Rethinking Bodies, Health, and Self-Care

Alive and Kicking

Sue Adstrum PhD

First published 2025 by Integrative Anatomy Solutions

Produced by Independent Ink
independentink.com.au

Copyright © Sue Adstrum PhD 2025

Cover design and internal illustrations by Daniela Catucci @ Catucci Design
Edited by Daina Lindeman
Internal design by Independent Ink
Typeset in Utopia Std by Post Pre-press Group, Brisbane
Image credits: page 3, public domain, https://commons.wikimedia.org/w/index. php?curid=29068101; page 29, image taken from Andreas Vesalius's De humani corporis fabrica (1543), page 174; page 29, anatomical studies of the shoulder by Leonardo da Vinci. Black chalk, pen and ink on paper; page 30, *On the Genealogy of Tissue Engineering and Regenerative Medicine*—scientific figure on ResearchGate. Available from: https://www. researchgate.net/figure/Mechanistic-physiology-GA-Borellis-De-Motu-Animalium-on-the-motion-of-animals_fig3_267730896 [accessed 8 Apr 2025]; page 89, Camille Flammarion, L'Atmosphère: Météorologie Populaire (Paris, 1888), pp. 163.

ISBN 978-0-473-74640-7 (paperback)
ISBN 978-0-473-74641-4 (epub)
ISBN 978-0-473-74642-1 (kindle)

Contents

For David, Benjamin, and Jonathan
With all my love.

Preface:
Rethinking Health, Rethinking the Body

"The world that we've made as a result of the level of thinking we have done thus far creates problems that we cannot solve at the same level as the level we created them. We cannot solve our problems with the same thinking we used when we created them."
—Albert Einstein

Healthcare is in crisis. Healthcare systems around the world are buckling under pressure. Patients wait too long. Professionals are burning out. Costs are spiralling. And many people feel increasingly disconnected from the very systems meant to care for them.

The cracks in modern healthcare are hard to ignore:

- Long waits and rushed appointments.
- Overworked professionals and chronic staff shortages.
- Patients searching Google for answers because they feel unheard.
- Healthcare workers walking away from work they once loved.
- Disjointed systems that struggle to treat the whole person.
- A mental health crisis that conventional systems can't keep up with.
- Environmental harm and unsustainable practices.
- Burnout, bureaucracy, and a growing sense of disconnection.

But this book isn't just about pointing out what's going wrong. It's about asking: "What if the real issue isn't just resourcing or infrastructure but also mindset?"

We've inherited a way of thinking that treats bodies like machines: breakable, replaceable, fixable in parts. But the human body isn't a machine. It's a living, sensing, adapting organism. And if we want healthier systems, we need to start by rethinking the way we understand the body at the centre of them.

Anatomy, the backbone of medicine, has often been taught in ways that divide and categorise. Muscles here. Organs there. A system at a time. But what happens when we view the body as a whole, alive, and context-sensitive? When we integrate science with story, biology with experience, tradition with innovation?

That's what this book explores.

I'm an integrative clinical anatomist. My background bridges clinical practice, academic research, and hands-on bodywork. Over the decades, I've come to believe that healing is more than procedures and prescriptions. It's about understanding. It's about connection.

This book isn't a textbook—and it's not a metaphysical manual either. It's a conversation—with ideas, with bodies, with history, and with you.

Written in everyday language, it welcomes readers of all backgrounds to stay curious. You'll meet patients, practitioners, and ideas that challenge convention. Each chapter brings a new lens for viewing health and wholeness.

You don't have to agree with everything. But if something stirs, unsettles, or opens a door—follow it.

Because healing our health systems begins with reimagining the bodies they're built around.

Let's start there. Together.

Navigation guide

This book unfolds as a layered exploration of what it means to have, care for, and understand a living human body. It begins by inviting readers to consider how perception, context, and personal experience shape our understanding of anatomy and health. From there, it traces the historical evolution of anatomical thinking—how we came to see bodies as dissected parts rather than as whole, sensing beings—and challenges that legacy by introducing fascia as a vital, yet long-overlooked, connective tissue system.

Through metaphors like the Living Wetsuit, the chapters offer accessible, fascia-aware ways to grasp structural integration, movement, pain, and healing. As the narrative builds, it deepens into broader reflections on embodiment, the mind-body connection, and culturally grounded models of wellbeing—like Te Whare Tapa Whā—that restore balance between physical, emotional, spiritual, and social health. Readers are invited to reflect not only on how we care for others but also how we care for ourselves. Practical chapters on self-care and self-treatment suggest small, empowering ways to reclaim agency in an overstretched system.

Ultimately, the book culminates in a call for change—not just in health policy or professional practice but in the very assumptions we hold about bodies, care, and healing. It offers a hopeful vision: that by reimagining the body as whole, alive, and contextually embedded, we can begin to co-create a more humane, sustainable, and fascia-aware future for healthcare—one breath, one body, one decision at a time.

Note on names

All names and identifying details in the stories I've shared about others throughout this book have been changed to protect the privacy of those involved.

Perception and Perspectives

"There are many realities. There are many versions of what may appear obvious. Whatever appears as the unshakeable truth, its exact opposite may be true in another context. After all, one's reality is but perception, viewed through various prisms of context."
—Amish Tripathi (2010)

Let's begin with a simple exercise.

Stand in front of a mirror. Hold up your hand with your palm facing you. Now, observe the reflection. Your real hand and its mirrored image look different. The reflection reveals details such as your fingernails, the wrinkles on your knuckles, and the tendons fanning beneath your skin. These differences are not illusions—they are two distinct perspectives of the same hand, the same reality.

Look at your hand through an X-ray or MRI scan, and yet another perspective emerges—this time from the inside out. A surgeon might see something different again. Each viewpoint reveals something valuable while concealing something else. No single perspective can capture the whole story of what your hand is or how it works.

Perception and perspective

Perspective is a key theme in this book, closely tied to two other concepts: *perception* and the act of *perceiving*. Together, these ideas shape how we experience, interpret, and understand the world—including our own bodies.

- **Perceive**—This is the act of becoming aware of our bodies through our senses—sight, touch, sound, smell, and taste. Some people also perceive the world through subtler senses, like intuition, interoception, and empathy.

- **Perception**—This is how our brain interprets what we observe. It is shaped by our experiences, knowledge, goals, and biases. One person may see the body as a fluid, breathing organism. Another may perceive it as a machine-like system of muscles, bones, and nerves. Others may view it as sacred, unknowable, or the dwelling place of spirit.

- **Perspective**—This is the angle or point of view we adopt. Like a window frame, perspective allows us to see certain things while hiding others.

We view everything through different lenses, and these help us make sense of what we perceive. Just as a hand can be seen directly, in a mirror, through a scan, or during surgery, the human body can be understood in multiple ways. Our perspectives are shaped by personal experience, education, culture, beliefs, and background. Each perspective adds depth and texture to our understanding of health and healthcare.

The house in the valley and the blind men with the elephant

Imagine a small cottage in a picturesque valley. It has four windows: one looks out over snow-capped mountains, another faces a tranquil river, the third reveals a dense forest, and the last opens toward farmland stretching towards a distant town. Each window offers a true view of the valley—but no single one shows it all.

Now think of the ancient parable of the blind men and the elephant. Six blind scholars, eager to understand what an elephant is, touch a different part of the animal. One feels an ear and says, "It's like a fan." Another touches a tusk: "A spear." The trunk: "A snake." The leg: "A tree." The side: "A wall." The tail: "A rope." Each one is convinced he has grasped the whole truth, but none have.

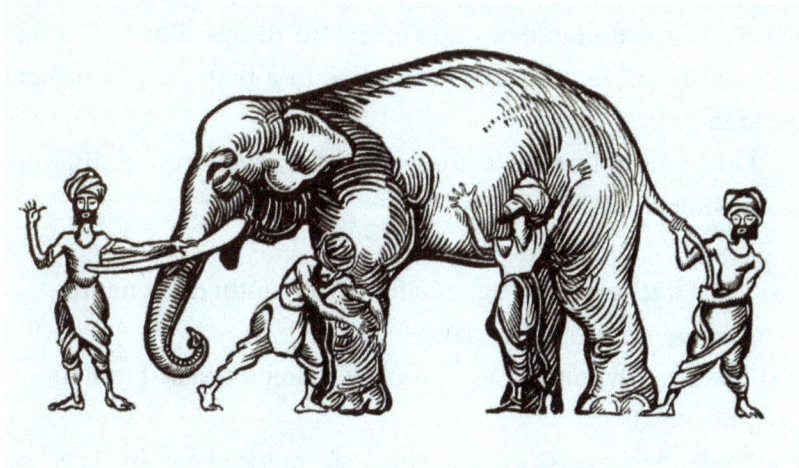

The blind men and the elephant

Each man describes the elephant based on the part he touches—an ear, a tusk, a leg—offering a partial truth shaped by limited experience. In the same way, different people (and disciplines) describe the body through their own lens. No single perspective captures the whole.

Each man's description is accurate in part—but limited. The elephant is all of these things and more. Their disagreement stems not from error but from incomplete information.

Both stories point to the same truth: multiple perspectives are needed to truly understand something complex—whether that's a hand, a valley, an elephant, or a human body. Like a disco ball reflecting light in many directions, each mirrored facet shows something real. When we step back and combine those views, a fuller picture starts to emerge.

Integrative anatomy

"Many views yield the truth ... after opposition has been expressed and softened, and all of the varying views have been brought into alignment ... so that all aspects of the truth are sung."
—Sherri Tepper (1989)

Today, most anatomists are scientists who study the human body using dissection, microscopy, or imaging. These methods give us clarity—but only through certain lenses. They help us measure structure, trace connections, and name things. But they don't necessarily tell us what it's like to live in a body, to feel or heal through it.

Other disciplines also study the body, each from a different angle. Their views are shaped by:

- Their **background** (e.g., anatomy, physiotherapy, neuro-science, anthropology, law).
- Their **motivation** (e.g., curiosity, career goals, funding priorities).
- Their **framework** (e.g., classical mechanics, history, complexity theory).
- Their **methods** (e.g., dissection, interviews, observation, interpretation).
- **Data collection and analysis methods.**
- Their **communication** style (e.g., technical papers, case studies, philosophical essays).

Each field sees something different. Yet researchers and clinicians often remain within their own silos, unaware of insights from other areas. Sometimes, this leads to disagreement about what's "correct". Other times, perspectives outside the dominant framework are ignored or dismissed altogether.

But if we begin to bring these views together—scientific, clinical, experiential, cultural—we start to see more. That's the heart of integrative anatomy. It doesn't claim one perspective is right and another wrong. Instead, it asks: *"What if all of them are useful?"*

Like shining multiple lights on a sculpture, each viewpoint illuminates new details. Together, they help us appreciate the body not just as a system of parts but as something more—living, layered, and whole.

An evolving change in perception— the lobster story

Our views can shift dramatically over time—even about what's edible, desirable, or respectable. A vivid example comes from a story that recently popped up in my LinkedIn feed:

> "In the 1700s, lobsters were so abundant in Massachusetts that they would wash up on beaches in piles two feet high. Back then, lobster was considered a cheap, low-class food— used as fertiliser or fed to prisoners and slaves. In fact, some indentured servants revolted when forced to eat lobster too often, and a law was passed a rule limiting them to no more than three lobster meals per week.
>
> When railroads expanded, train crews began serving lobster to passengers. Unaware of its reputation, travellers from other states assumed it was a delicacy. Demand grew. Perception shifted. And lobster transformed from poor man's fare to a luxury symbol of affluence."

It's a great example of how supply chains, marketing, and context shape perception. But I can't help wondering: what would a lobster say about this retelling? Or the workers who harvested them in harsh conditions? Or the women who had to prepare and cook them daily?

This simple story reminds us: context changes meaning. What once seemed unimportant or undesirable can become revered. And the same is true for anatomy. Over time, ideas once dismissed—like fascia, subtle energy, or lived experience—can become vital pieces of a bigger puzzle.

Changing how we see the body

The lobster anecdote isn't just a quirky aside—it's a preview of what's to come. Perceptions of the body are just as vulnerable to trends, biases, and blind spots as any other human idea. But when we step back and consider, new possibilities emerge.

This is what this book invites you to do: take a fresh look. Examine old ideas from new angles. Question what you've been taught—and listen to your own lived experience, too.

Has there been a moment in your life—perhaps a conversation, a book, or even a quiet realisation—that shifted how you see the body, health, or healing? Something that nudged your perspective, even just a little?

You don't need to have an answer. But stay curious. Sometimes the most meaningful insights begin as gentle questions.

This book offers one such question: *"What if we have been seeing the body through an imperfect lens?"* What if, instead of a machine made of separate physical parts, it's a living, sensing **human matrix**—a dynamic field of physical and energetic elements that shape how we heal, move, and feel?

Anatomised Bodies

02

"The Church says: the body is a sin.
Science says: the body is a machine.
Advertising says: the body is a business.
The body says: I am a fiesta."
—Eduardo Galeano (1997)

What is a body, really?

We all have one—but if you had to explain what a body *is* to someone else, how would you begin? Whether they know you well or not, putting the body into words isn't always straightforward.

Every human life depends on having a living body. While there are universal similarities, each body is also unique, irreplaceable, and invaluable. We often refer to "the body" as a whole, yet when it is dissected or studied, it appears to be made up of many distinct parts. Adding to the mystery, the body is constantly changing—from the moment of conception to the end of life. The body you had as a child looked different to the one you have now, and even different from the one you had last year—yet it's still *your* body.

Throughout history, human bodies have been understood in different ways. This is reflected in how they've been depicted in art, medicine, and philosophy across cultures and eras—from ancient Egypt, Greece, and India to Renaissance Italy, Ming Dynasty China, and more modern multicultural societies. Even today, acupuncturists, brain surgeons, massage therapists, and internal medicine physicians use slightly different, yet overlapping, anatomical frameworks—each aligned with their approach to care.

Writers, artists, scientists, and scholars have described the body from many angles, shaped by the medical knowledge, tools, and cultural assumptions of their time. Like beams of light bouncing off a mirrored disco ball, each perspective reveals a facet of the body's wholeness that might otherwise have gone unnoticed. The more perspectives we include—both individually and collectively—the better we understand what a body truly *is*.

Our thinking about the body's structure has been shaped by centuries of observation, study, and interpretation. As a result, there isn't one single way to define the body—there are many. Here are just a few dictionary definitions:

- A tangible, physical form.
- A person's mortal form, distinct from their soul or consciousness.
- A lifeless body (a corpse or cadaver).
- A collection of organs, tissues, cells, and molecules.
- The main (central) part of a person's body, distinct from the limbs and the head.
- The "important" parts of a person's body—without those deemed less significant (like fascia).
- A biologically whole structure that functions as an organised unit.
- A living structure that is influenced by—and influences—more than just its physical form.
- A person.

You may find that some of these definitions resonate more than others. That's okay. Different perspectives make sense to different people at different times. Anatomical understanding isn't fixed—it evolves over centuries, and even within a single lifetime. And if we want to care well for our bodies and wellbeing, expanding how we think about the body can be a good place to begin.

Anatomy

"Anatomists say: the body is our reason for being."
—Sue Adstrum (2021)

I'm a university-qualified clinical anatomist (among other things)—someone who studies and describes the structure of the human body. The word *anatomy* comes from the Greek *anatomia*, meaning "cutting up" or "dissection". Anatomists study the body by breaking it down—both physically and conceptually—to better understand its structure and how it works. While many people picture an anatomist with a scalpel, the work actually happens in two main ways:

1. **Mental dissection**—The human body is astonishingly complex—perhaps too complex to fully grasp in one go. So, anatomists conceptually divide it into smaller, more manageable parts. This makes it easier to study and describe. But it can also encourage a more depersonalised view—reducing the body to diagrams, labels, or cadavers, rather than recognising it as a living, feeling whole.

2. **Physical dissection**—This involves cutting into a chemically preserved cadaver to reveal its internal structures—lungs, tendons, thyroid glands, and so on. Contrary to popular belief, sharp tools are often less important than blunt ones—including the anatomist's fingers—when used to gently separate tissue layers.

Have you ever noticed your understanding of the body shift—subtly or dramatically—after an experience, a class, an illness, or a healing moment? What changed in how you related to your own body afterward?

Both methods aim to make sense of the body by breaking it down. Without these techniques, we'd struggle to describe its parts. Over time, this work has led to the identification of thousands of anatomical structures—and new discoveries are still emerging as technology advances.

ORGANISM	A whole and alive person's body
ORGAN SYSTEM	A group of organs that work together to perform a particular set of body functions (e.g. muscular system)
ORGAN	A body part that performs a specific function (e.g. a muscle)
TISSUE	A group of cells that have a similar structure and function together as a unit (e.g. muscle tissue)
CELL	The smallest biological unit (e.g. a muscle cell)

A brief history of anatomy in Western thought

Ancient roots

Western anatomy traces back to ancient Greece. Early philosophers like Alcmaeon of Croton (5th century BCE) made foundational anatomical observations—such as noting that the eyes are connected to the brain. Hippocrates (c. 460–370 BCE), often called the "Father of Medicine", encouraged systematic observation over supernatural explanations.

Herophilus and Erasistratus, working in Alexandria around 300 BCE, were among the first to perform human anatomical dissections. Their research advanced medical understanding, though there were rumours they may also have dissected living prisoners (as well as cadavers).

Galen's legacy

During the Roman Empire, Galen of Pergamon (129–c. 216 CE) became the most influential anatomist of the time. Roman law prohibited human dissection, so Galen relied heavily on animal studies. His observations, although limited by today's standards, dominated anatomical thought for more than 1,500 years.

The Renaissance revival

In medieval Europe, much anatomical knowledge was preserved by Islamic and Indian scholars. In Europe, dissection remained rare until the 12th century, when universities began to allow the dissection of a small number of executed criminals each year. By the 14th century, public dissections became highly ritualised, multi-day events, often in winter to delay decay.

These dissections were typically performed by a three-person team:

- The **professor** (or *lector*), who sat in an elevated chair far from the cadaver, reading from a Latin textbook (usually Galen's writings).
- The **sector** (usually a barber-surgeon), who carried out the dissection.
- The **ostensor** (or demonstrator), who used a rod to point to the anatomical structures being read aloud about.

The goal wasn't discovery—it was demonstration. These performances were designed to illustrate and reinforce Galen's teachings, not challenge them. That's why Andreas Vesalius's decision to dissect cadavers himself, teach from what he observed, and correct Galenic errors was so revolutionary.

In the 1500s, Vesalius laid the foundation for modern anatomy by insisting that knowledge should come from direct observation—not inherited texts.

Technology transforms the view

The 19th and 20th centuries brought huge change. Formalin improved cadaver preservation. X-rays, MRIs, and CT scans allowed us to look inside the living body without making an incision. Today, 3D modelling, virtual dissection tables, and AI-assisted scans continue to transform how we explore and teach anatomy.

Branches of anatomy

Over time, anatomists have developed specialised ways of exploring the body's structure. Each branch focuses on different aspects of what makes us human—from the visible to the microscopic, from embryonic development to evolutionary comparison. When these perspectives are combined, they offer a far more complete view than any one approach alone.

GROSS ANATOMY The study of body parts you can see without a microscope	Surface anatomy	Looking at body features on the outside
	Systemic anatomy	Studying the body one system at a time (like the nervous or muscular system)
	Regional anatomy	Focusing on a specific area of the body (like the shoulder or pelvis)
	Clinical anatomy	Understanding the body in ways that help with diagnosing and treating injuries and illness
	Surgical anatomy	Understanding the body in ways that help during surgery
MICROSCOPIC ANATOMY The study of tiny structures you need a microscope to see	Organology	The study of organs
	Histology	The study of tissues
	Cytology	The study of cells
	Structural biology	The study of how very small biological structures are built
RADIOLOGICAL ANATOMY	Studying the body using scans like X-rays or MRIs	
DEVELOPMENTAL ANATOMY	Looking at how the body grows and changes before birth	
BIOLOGICAL (OR PHYSICAL) ANTHROPOLOGY	Studying how human bodies change, adapt, and evolve across different environments and historical periods	
COMPARATIVE ANATOMY	Comparing human bodies with animals to see what's similar or different	
INTEGRATIVE ANATOMY	Bringing together ideas from different fields to understand the body as a whole	

Why anatomy matters

"Anatomy serves as the handmaid to the art of the physician and to the craft of the surgeon." —Professor Edward Barclay-Smith (1922)

Anatomy underpins everything in medicine. It's the starting point for understanding how the body functions (physiology), what happens when things go wrong (pathology), and how we treat or support healing. Whether you're a healthcare professional, a student, or simply someone trying to care for yourself, keeping your anatomical understanding fresh and accurate matters.

Anatomy matters because our understanding of the body shapes how we think about health and medicine. It is the foundation upon which all other aspects of healthcare are built—and the more we know, the better we can care for ourselves and others. This is illustrated in the following story.

STRUCTURE
ANATOMY

↕

FUNCTION
PHYSIOLOGY
PATHOLOGY

↕

HEALTH CARE
& REMEDIAL
TREATMENT

Understanding the body's structure helps us explain how it works, what happens to it when it's injured or unwell, and what can be done to improve its health.

An exercise in clinical anatomy

My deeper dive into fascia-focused anatomy and health care began—unexpectedly—while I was studying public health. I read paper after paper on clinical conditions and treatment outcomes. But not one of them mentioned fascia.

It was like the fascia had disappeared.

My clinical experience told me a different story. Hands-on, the body felt like an interconnected whole. But the literature I read kept breaking it into parts. That disconnect became a spark.

This prompted me to move from public health into the anatomy department and began a research master's degree. I didn't just want a new qualification—I wanted the language to describe what my hands already knew.

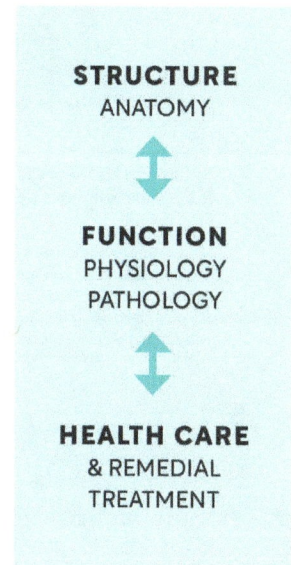

My supervisor suggested I study the transverse humeral ligament (THL). I'd never heard of it. It sounded obscure. But sometimes the smallest structures open the biggest doors.

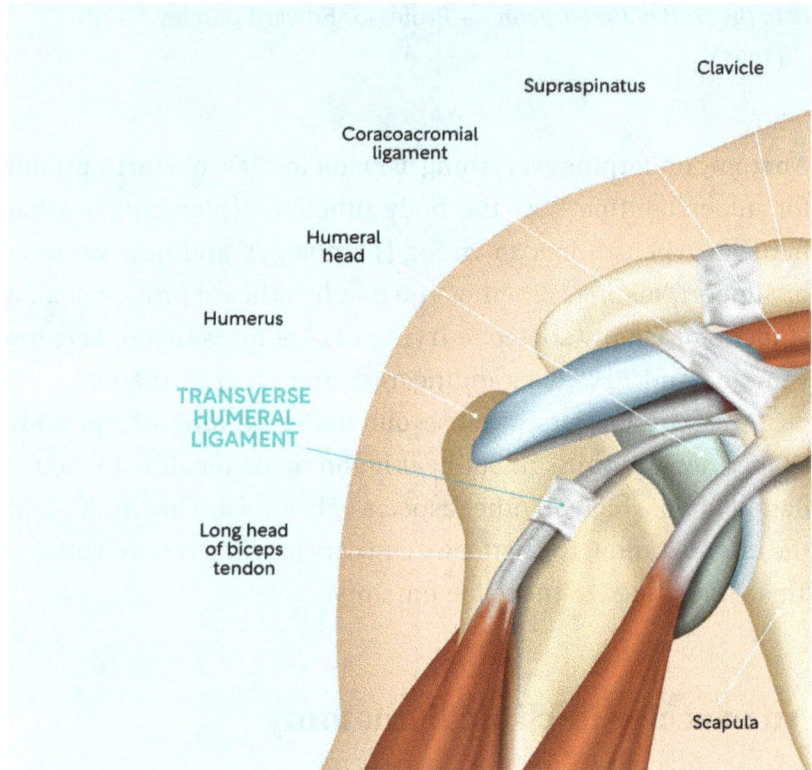

Like any good researcher, I started in the library. The THL had little coverage. Gross anatomy described it as a fibrous band spanning the intertubercular sulcus (a groove in the humerus bone), stabilising the long head of the biceps brachii tendon (LBT). Its function was vaguely acknowledged—an injury could cause instability and dislocation. But I wanted to know more.

To better understand the THL, I needed to examine it from multiple perspectives—from the front, the sides, and deep inside its structure. This meant applying four different anatomical and histological techniques—most of which were new to me. A steep learning curve lay ahead, but I was up for the challenge.

What followed was a deep, multi-method investigation—working with plastinated slices, performing detailed dissections, analysing tissue microscopically, and even attempting immuno-histochemical staining. There were moments of awe, frustration (including one lab mix-up that destroyed some of my final specimens), and discovery.

The big surprise? The so-called ligament may not be a ligament at all. It appeared to be an extension of the subscapularis tendon—more like a tendon expansion than a bone-to-bone connector.

Microscopic analysis revealed densely packed collagen fibres, a few nerve endings, and hints of proprioceptive function. I realised it wasn't just stabilising the tendon—it might also be helping the brain sense shoulder position and movement.

For me, this journey confirmed what I'd felt all along: the body is more interconnected, subtle, and intelligent than we often give it credit for. And sometimes, even the smallest structures invite us to rethink everything we thought we knew.

Have you ever encountered something in your work, study, or personal experience that challenged a long-held assumption? How did it shift your understanding?

Fascia

03

"[Fascia] sheathes, permeates, divides and sub-divides every portion of all animal bodies; surrounding and penetrating every muscle and all its fibers—every artery, and every fiber and principle thereto belonging."
—Andrew Taylor Still (1899)

For centuries, Western medicine has relied on dissecting human cadavers to understand the body. This process involves carefully cutting a whole body into lots of smaller, examinable-sized pieces—separating the lungs, heart, muscles, bones, and brain. As a result, the body has often been described as if it were a complex machine made up of separate, individual "parts". A good example of this is the "musculoskeletal system", which envisions muscles, bones, tendons, and ligaments as distinct components working together to produce movement.

While this perspective has been incredibly useful, it doesn't tell the whole story. One essential but often overlooked "body part" isn't really a part at all—it's fascia. Fascia is a vast, three-dimensional web of soft connective tissue that weaves through and around everything under the skin, integrating every structure in the body.

Fascia doesn't just hold things together—it allows them all to glide freely without friction. It also plays a key role in nearly every bodily process, from cell communication to healing and recovery. In fact, all of the body's physiological and communications systems depend on fascia, and disruptions in this network are often linked to pain, mobility issues, and other health challenges.

Fascia is a word that gets thrown around a lot these days, but what does it actually mean? In the simplest terms, it refers to the body's soft connective tissue—the stuff that wraps, supports, and holds everything together. But, as you'll shortly find out, it is far more interesting than that!

Discovering my passion for fascia

You're not alone if you've never heard of fascia. For the first 20 years of my career as a physiotherapist in New Zealand, I had only a vague awareness of fascia as some isolated bits of tissue—but I knew almost nothing about fascia itself. It wasn't in our textbooks, never came up in lectures, and wasn't a topic of discussion among colleagues or at professional seminars. It simply didn't exist in my medical world—yet, as I would later discover, it is an extremely important part of our bodies.

My introduction to fascia wasn't through research or formal training, but through something more personal: pain. In the early 1980s, I was struggling with persistent neck and back issues. The standard treatments of the time—bed rest, foam collars, hot packs, joint mobilisation, exercises, and medication—provided temporary relief, but nothing lasting. I wanted something more.

That's when a chance encounter changed everything. I met a visiting Structural Integration practitioner who spoke about fascia in a way I'd never heard before. I was intrigued—but only just. My focus was on the relief I felt from her fascia-based hands-on therapy, not the structure she was working with. Still, that meeting planted a seed. It led me to explore fascia-relating treatment methods, eventually taking me to San Francisco and then to Maui, where I studied craniosacral therapy.

Then something extraordinary happened.

After finishing a class in Maui, I took a walk through the lush 'Iao Valley State Monument. The air was thick with the scent of damp earth, and towering ancient trees cast dappled light over a tumbling stream. As I followed the winding path, something shifted. I had what I can only describe as a tutorial—not a vision in the traditional sense, but a deep, wordless knowing.

I watched the water flow over moss-covered rocks in thin, white veils and suddenly saw fascia in a way I never had before. I "saw" that fascia is like the flowing white sheets of water that streamed over the moss-edged rocks. It was not just tissue, but a flowing interconnected system—essential to the body's function and health. I didn't hear words, but I walked away with a certainty: fascia was important. More than that, it was going to be my work.

For someone who had never considered herself particularly "woo-woo", this experience was a wake-up call. It wasn't until years later that I came across a passage from Andrew Taylor Still (the founder of osteopathy) that perfectly captured what I had glimpsed in that valley:

"The soul of man with all the streams of pure living water seems to dwell in the fascia of his body." —Andrew Taylor Still (1899)

From that moment on, I was all in. I immersed myself in studying and practising fascia-relating bodywork—craniosacral therapy, myofascial release, and more. As a physiotherapist, I was fascinated by the results I was seeing, especially in conditions not typically treated with manual therapy. Asthma, chronic pain, post-traumatic stress, birth injuries, digestive issues, even neurological disorders—patients with these conditions were experiencing improvements, sometimes dramatic ones.

Yet, despite these successes, I faced a challenge. I couldn't explain why fascia-focused treatments worked in the scientific terms my profession valued. Worse, when I tried, my enthusiasm was often met with scepticism—or outright dismissal. If I was going to introduce this work to my colleagues, I needed to understand it on a deeper level.

So, I did something unexpected—I went back to university. As a "mature student", I studied everything from anatomy and anthropology to medical history and public health, weaving together a transdisciplinary perspective that shaped the way I now teach, write, and think about health-care.

That journey—sparked by pain and a moment of insight in a Hawaiian valley—has led me to a lifelong mission: helping others understand the vital role of fascia in health and wellbeing. And I've never looked back.

A very brief history of fascia

The word itself likely comes from the ancient Greek *taenia* (ταινία), which described long, thin, ribbon-like objects. The Romans later borrowed it as *fascia*, using it to describe all sorts of things: bandages, headbands, sashes, strips of land, and even certain types of long, slender fish. Today, *fascia* pops up in some unexpected places—it can refer to the front panel on a mobile phone, the bold stripes on a bird's feathers, or even the web of intangible connections between people and their surroundings (Murray, 2009).

In the world of medicine, *fascia* first appeared in English language writing in 1615, when anatomist Helkiah Crooke described the body's "almost infinite" number of membranes. But for nearly two centuries, the word was more often linked to surgical bandages than body tissue—hence terms like *fascia spiralis* (a spiral roller bandage) and *fascia tortilis* (a type of tourniquet).

It wasn't until the 19th and 20th centuries that fascia started gaining real attention in anatomy. New preservation techniques kept cadavers from decomposing too quickly, allowing anatomists to study soft tissue in more detail. But there was a catch—these preservation fluids (often containing alcohol and formaldehyde) dried out the fascia, making it stiff, thick, and opaque.

For a more in-depth discussion of this topic, see Adstrum (2021, 2022) and Adstrum & Nicholson (2019)]

This was both a blessing and a curse. On one hand, it allowed researchers to identify new fascial structures (Warwick & Williams, 1973). On the other, the dried-out fascia obscured everything underneath it, making it difficult to see muscles, blood vessels, nerves, and organs. Frustrated anatomists began routinely cutting away and discarding it during dissections—a process known as "cleaning the body". Over time, this habit led to fascia being largely ignored—not just by medical students, but by entire generations of doctors, physiotherapists, health researchers, and educators. In fact, most people outside of the medical field had never even heard of it.

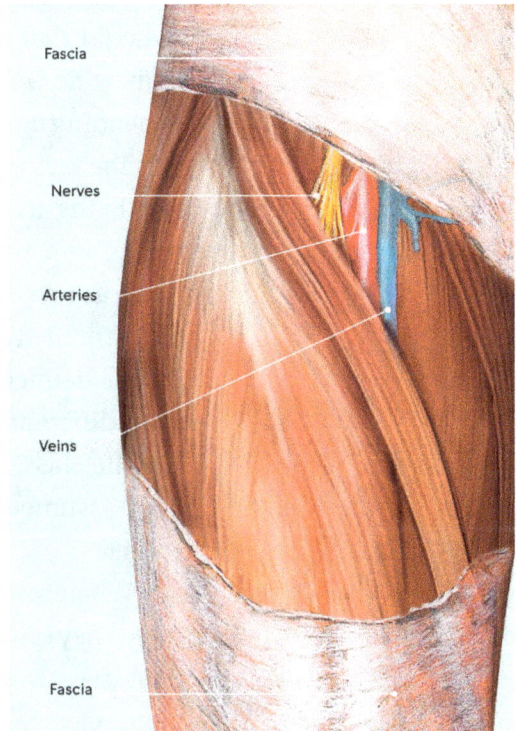

Fascia
Nerves
Arteries
Veins
Fascia

Before and after anatomical 'cleaning'

This artwork gives a fascinating peek beneath the skin surface! It illustrates how the muscles of the trunk and thighs—along with nerves (yellow), arteries (red), and veins (blue)—appear before and after their natural covering of delicate, gauzy white fascia is carefully removed ("cleaned away") during anatomical dissection.

What do you mean, fascia?

"There has been a paradigm shift in how fascia is known. The old way of describing fascia was someone opening up the body from the outside and showing all of the layers. We now know there are no layers or spaces. Everything is continuous. We now see the whole, vibrating fascial web." —Professor Carol Davis, British Fascia Symposium (2020)

At the start of the 21st century, something began to shift. Fascia, once a niche topic mostly of interest to anatomists and surgeons, suddenly became a hot topic across many fields. Scientists, clinicians, and researchers from diverse backgrounds were now studying it—and they weren't all on the same page about what fascia actually was.

Was it a distinct piece of tissue that could be dissected? The material that made up those dissectible structures? Or was it a body-wide web of soft tissue that varied in texture and function depending on its role?

The lack of a clear, agreed-upon definition meant that *fascia* was being used to describe all three—sometimes as a type of tissue, sometimes as a specific anatomical structure, and sometimes as an entire body system. The confusion only deepened as different medical dictionaries, anatomy textbooks, and scientific papers defined it in their own ways. Different professions—and even different countries—had their own interpretations, much like the classic tale of the blind scholars describing an elephant. Each assumed their own experience was the whole truth. But it wasn't.

When researchers realised what was happening, alarm bells rang. They saw that this inconsistency was creating a communications mess, making it harder for people to understand and discuss fascia clearly (Adstrum et al., 2017). For scientists, healthcare professionals, and anatomists alike, precision matters. Every anatomical term needs to refer to a single, clearly defined structure—otherwise confusion reigns.

To help solve the problem, fascia researchers introduced two new anatomical terms: *a fascia* (referring to a specific structure) and *the fascial system* (referring to the broader network). This small but significant distinction helped people be more precise when talking about fascia.

Still, the conversation isn't over. Some people continue to view fascia through different lenses, and debate continues over how best to define it. But the introduction of clearer terminology has at least given researchers and clinicians a common starting point.

TERM	GENERAL MEANING	FORMAL DEFINITION
Fascia	All of the body's soft connective tissue parts	A non-specific word that anatomists apply to "sheaths, sheets, or other dissectible masses of connective tissue that are large enough to be visible to the unaided eye as well as the tissue from which they are composed" (Standring, 2016).
Fascial tissue	Soft connective tissue	Connective tissue proper.
A fascia (plural, fasciae)	A distinct and dissectible piece of fascial tissue	"A sheath, a sheet or any number of dissectible aggregations of connective tissue that forms beneath the skin to attach, enclose, separate muscles and other internal organs" (Stecco & Schleip, 2016).
The fascial system	A body-pervading web of fascial tissue	"The three-dimensional continuum of soft, collagen containing loose and dense fibrous connective tissue that permeates the body. It incorporates elements such as adipose tissue, adventitia and neurovascular sheaths, aponeuroses, deep and superficial fasciae, epineurium, joint capsules, ligaments, membranes, meninges, myofascial expansions, periosteum, retinacula, septa, tendons, visceral fasciae, and all the intramuscular and intermuscular connective tissues including endo-/peri-/epimysium. The fascial system surrounds, interweaves, and blends with muscles, bones, nerves, blood vessels, and internal organs, creating a functional, integrated environment that enables all body systems to operate in an integrated manner" (Adstrum et al., 2017; & Stecco et al., 2018).

Fascial tissue

Fascia is usually classified as a type of soft connective tissue that assumes a variety of forms—ranging from delicate sacs and membranes to tough, fibrous sheets, cords, bands, or ropes. Rather than existing as a single uniform structure, fascia weaves through and between the body's other parts, seamlessly shifting from one form to another, and uniquely adapting to the moment-by-moment functional demands placed on it.

At its core, fascial tissue is a living matrix—a network of hydrated ground substance threaded with different types of cells and structural protein fibers.

Fascial vocabulary

Until recently, the word 'fascia' was used to describe several overlapping anatomical concepts, leading to confusion in its understanding. To clarify this, fascia researchers developed a system to distinguish between the different meanings and uses of this term (Adstrum et al.,. 2017).

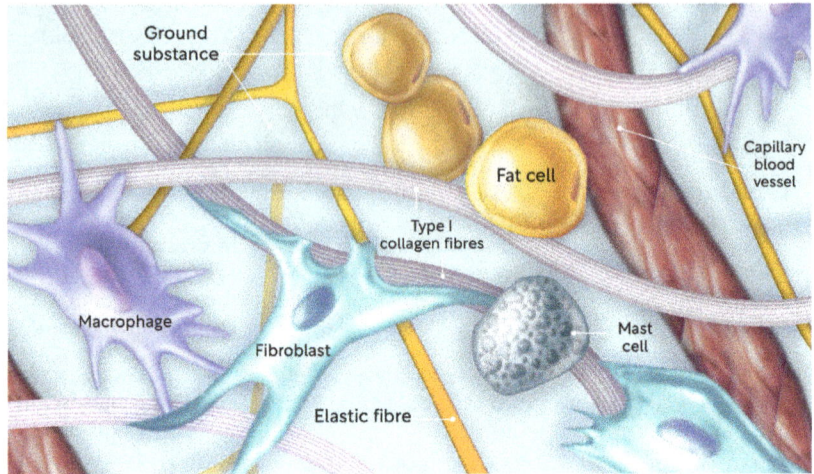

Fascial tissue contains a mix of cells and fibres suspended in a jelly-like ground substance. In some areas, it's much denser — packed with strong collagen fibres — and has fewer cells, because most of the space is taken up by those fibres.

Ground substance

Fat cell

Capillary blood vessel

Type I collagen fibres

Macrophage

Mast cell

Fibroblast

Elastic fibre

The most abundant—and least discussed—component of fascia is its ground substance. Essentially jellified water, it ranges from sticky to fluid depending on its location and conditions. Interestingly, when its surface is broken—by pulling it apart or piercing it with a scalpel—the gel collapses almost instantly into a fragile web of filaments. This disrupted form, often called areolar tissue, gets its name from the unnatural spaces (areolae) that appear between its lattice of threads.

In its natural, living state, fascia's ground substance is transparent and largely featureless—at least under an ordinary microscope. Without advanced imaging techniques like those used by Benias et al. (2019), it mostly escapes visual detection. And because traditional anatomical, histological, and surgical methods tend to dry it out, damage it, or remove it altogether, it has historically often been overlooked in scientific descriptions. Instead, attention has typically focused on fascia's more visually striking components—its fibres and cells.

In many parts of the body, fascia's ground substance is densely reinforced with structural proteins that give it strength and elasticity. The most common of these, type I collagen fibres, are incredibly strong, white in colour, and visible to the naked eye.

However, contrary to many textbook descriptions, these fibres only appear in places where the tissue needs extra tensile strength to withstand stretching and pulling without tearing. Meanwhile, elastin fibres—true to their name—allow fascia to stretch and recoil, adapting elastically to the movements of underlying structures such as the lungs or contracting muscles.

Fascia also contains a diverse mix of cells, whose types and numbers shift according to the tissue's needs at any given time. All of these cells are suspended in—and often move through—the ground substance. Fibroblasts, the main cell type, are responsible for producing and maintaining the gel-fibre (extracellular) matrix. Some areas also contain fat cells (adipocytes), while immune cells like macrophages and mast cells are recruited when needed. In injured or diseased tissue, you may even find red and white blood cells, bacteria, fungi, or cancer cells.

Far from being a passive wrapping material, fascia is a dynamic living matrix—constantly adapting, responding, and changing in ways that science is only beginning to fully appreciate.

What makes fascia so special?

"The fascial system surrounds, infuses with, and has potential to influence profoundly every muscle, bone, nerve, blood vessel, organ, and cell of the body. Fascia also separates, supports, connects, and protects everything. This three-dimensional web of connective tissue is alive and ever changing as the body demands. Thus it is a network for information exchange, influencing and influenced by every structure, system, and cell in the organism. Like air and gravity, its influence is so all-pervasive that we have tended to take it for granted." —John F Barnes (1990)

Note: If you'd like a deeper dive into fascia—how it works, what it does, and why it matters—I've explored it in more detail in my previous book, *The Living Wetsuit.*

Fascia just isn't some background tissue holding everything together—it's a dynamic, body-wide network of tissue that shapes, supports, and connects *everything* inside you. What it's made of— its mix of cells, fibres, and gel-like ground substance—determines its qualities (how it behaves) and functions (what it actually does).

For over 200 years, the only people who really paid attention to it were anatomists and surgeons. And from their perspective, it seemed like a tough, fibrous wrapping that simply *covered, contained, separated,* and *filled gaps* between what were considered the body's more important structures, like muscles, blood vessels, organs, and nerves. In other words, it was seen as useful but not particularly interesting.

That view has changed—dramatically. Thanks to a surge in interest from all kinds of disciplines, we now know that fascia is *far* more than just packaging. It's a three-dimensional, living web that unites everything inside you. It holds things in place, protects them from harm, and plays a vital role in how your body develops, moves, heals, and even communicates with itself.

Because fascia is everywhere, no part of your body exists—or works—in isolation. If you think of your body as a symphony, fascia is the conductor—helping everything stay in tune and work together.

And that, as some like to say, is pretty *fascia*-nating.

"Fascia is a cacophony of functions and information ... The fascial system supports, protects, evolves and connects the human body."
—Bordoni & Simonelli (2018)

The Musculoskeletal Body Machine

04

"The musculoskeletal body machine is an interconnected system of bones, muscles, ligaments, tendons, and nerves that work together to support the body's posture and movement—like a well-designed machine." —ChatGPT

For centuries, the musculoskeletal body (a classic example of an anatomised body model) has been at the heart of medicine, sports, and rehabilitation. Healthcare professionals such as doctors, surgeons, physiotherapists, massage therapists, and fitness trainers work with it daily to treat injuries, improve movement, and increase strength. When these experts talk about the musculoskeletal system, they're essentially referring to the way they view the body.

At first, "musculoskeletal" might sound like a mix of muscles (musculo) and bones (skeletal), but it actually includes more than that. It also involves tendons, joints, cartilage, ligaments, and even the nervous system—the brain, spinal cord, and nerves that control movement, pain perception, and overall function. Because of this, it's more accurate to think of the musculoskeletal system as a *neuro-musculo-skeletal system*.

From the typical musculoskeletal perspective, the body is often seen as:

- A tangible, physical form
- A person's mortal form, separate from their soul or consciousness
- A collection of the body's big, obvious structures—muscles, bones, and nerves—with things like fascia often being overlooked

This way of seeing the body can limit our understanding of its full potential in both health and dysfunction. It's just one way of viewing the body, and it restricts the types of treatments available to those seeking help.

The evolution of the musculoskeletal model

Our understanding of the musculoskeletal system began to take shape during the European Renaissance. Before this period, medicine was based on the humoral theory—the idea that health depends on the balance of four vital body fluids: blood, phlegm, black bile, and yellow bile. Ancient thinkers like Hippocrates, Aristotle, and Galen believed that health problems, including pain, were caused by imbalances in these fluids. Treatments like bloodletting, purging, or dietary changes were used to restore balance.

Physicians at the time focused on understanding organs (like the liver and spleen), fluid-carrying vessels (like arteries and veins), and membranes (like the peritoneum and pleura), which they believed regulated the body's humoral balance. As a result, anatomists concentrated on the body's abdomen, chest, and head, with muscles receiving little attention.

That began to change during the Renaissance. Pioneers emerged, such as:

- **Andreas Vesalius** (1514–1564), whose dissections and anatomical drawings provided accurate depictions of the body's bones and muscles, and
- **Leonardo da Vinci** (1452–1519), who used his knowledge of anatomy to create lifelike art and study how the body moved, played a key role in shifting anatomical focus from static organs to the muscles and bones responsible for movement.

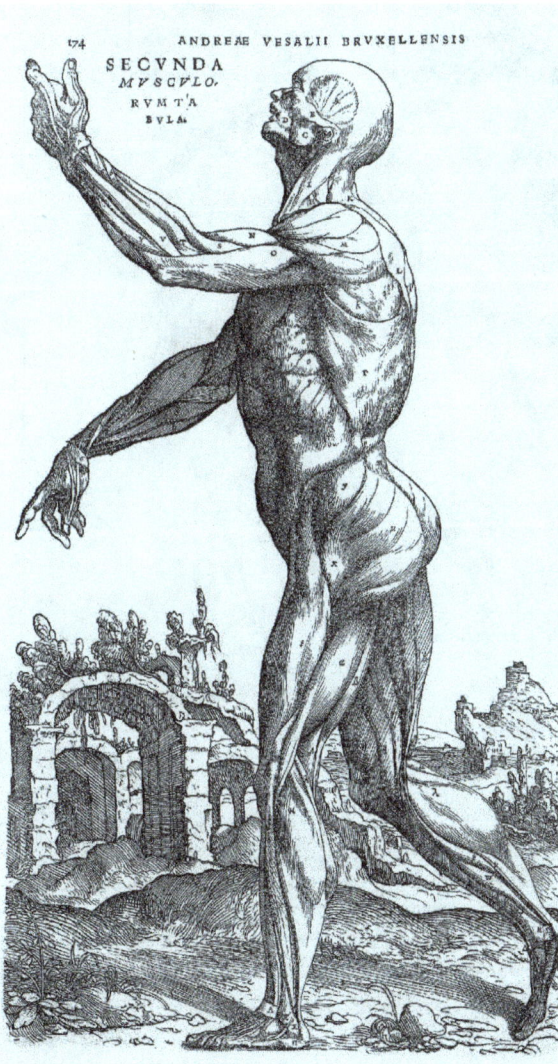

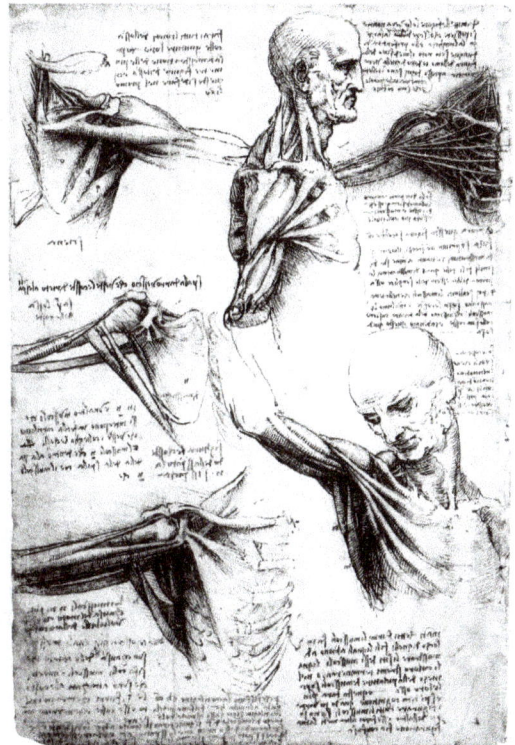

Andreas Vesalius and Leonardo da Vinci anatomical drawings

Left: Andreas Vesalius' dissections and anatomical drawings provided accurate depictions of the body's bones and muscles.

Right: Leonardo da Vinci's lifelike art played key roles in shifting anatomical focus from static organs to the muscles and bones responsible for movement

This functional approach was further expanded by **Giovanni Alfonso Borelli** (1608–1679), who applied Galileo's principles of mechanics to understand how muscles and bones work together to produce movement, comparing the body to a machine—a system of levers.

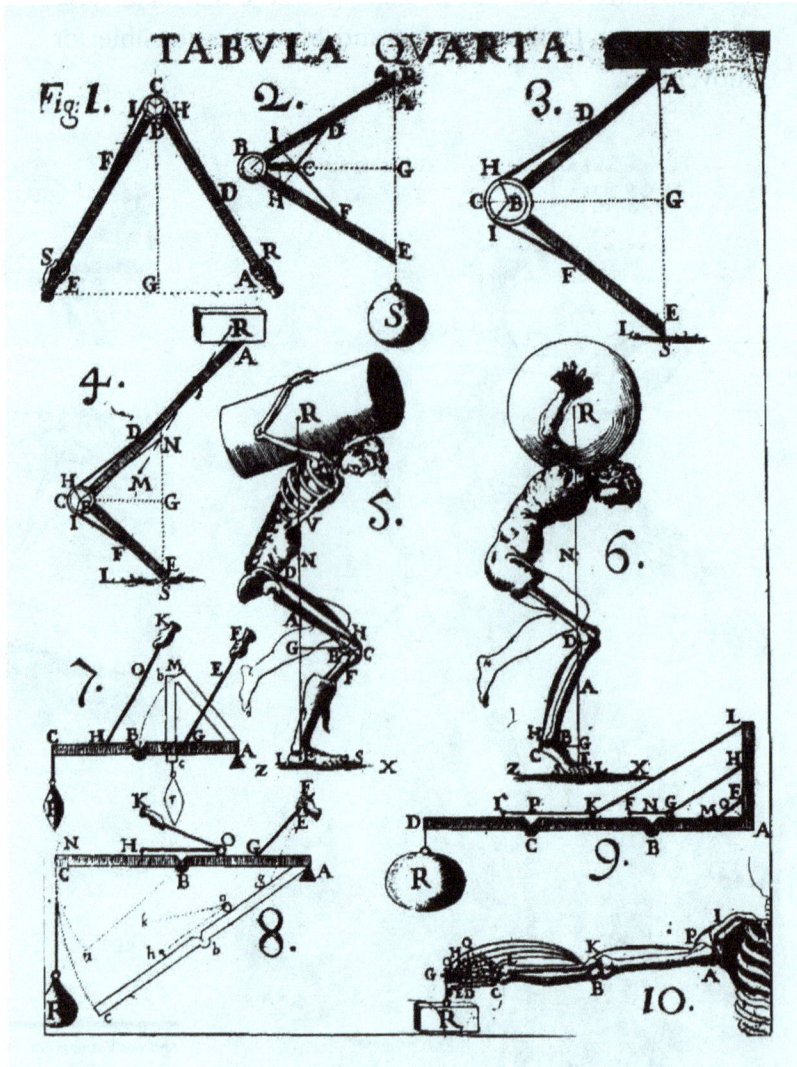

TABVLA QVARTA.

Explaining body movement

Scientists have long tried to understand how the body moves, and their answers depend on how they view the body's structure. These differing perspectives have led to the development of different models. One of the oldest and most popular is the **biomechanical model**, which sees the body as a system of levers. In this view, bones are rigid bars, joints are pivot points, and muscles provide the force to move them.

Muscles contract and pull on bones through tendons, causing movement. This model is great for explaining activities like lifting heavy objects or performing precise, powerful actions, such as a ballerina dancing on tiptoe or a pitcher throwing a fastball.

But there's also a newer model gaining attention: the **biotensegrity model**. This model views the body as a unified whole, where fascia (the connective tissue) holds everything together and influences movement. Unlike the biomechanical model, which breaks the body into parts, biotensegrity sees the body as an interconnected system.

The term **tensegrity**—short for tensional integrity—was coined by architect and systems theorist Buckminster Fuller to describe a structural system made of solid struts (which resist compression) and tensioned cables (which maintain the structure's shape and stability). The parts are held together by a continuous balance of tension and compression. No part functions in isolation. Apply pressure to one part of a tensegrity structure, and the entire form shifts to adapt.

Applying this concept to biology, orthopaedic surgeon Stephen Levin proposed **biotensegrity** as a new way to explain body movement and structure. In this model, the body's form and function are maintained not by stacking parts like bricks but through a dynamic, responsive balance of tension (mainly fascia) and compression (bones). Movement is a whole-body event—an orchestrated change in shape, not just a matter of muscle force.

Lever = the arm and forearm bones (humerus, radius, and ulna);

Fulcrum = the elbow joint where these bones meet;

Load = the weight of the forearm bones, surrounding tissues, and anything else being moved;

Effort = the pulling force of a muscle, transmitted through its tendon into the bone.

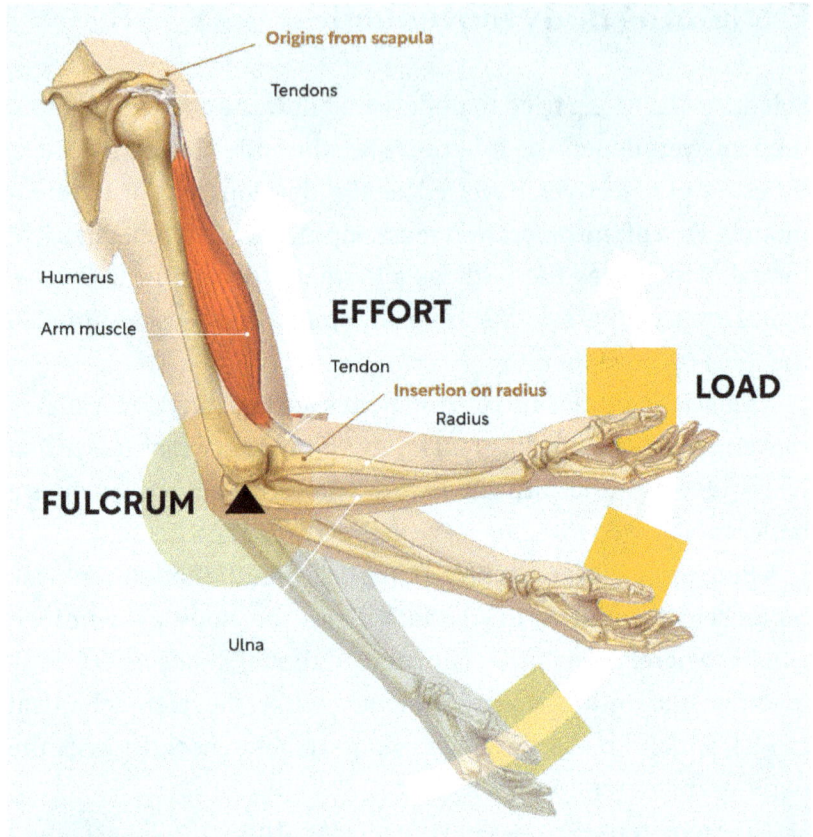

Origins from scapula

Tendons

Humerus

Arm muscle

EFFORT

Tendon

Insertion on radius

Radius

LOAD

FULCRUM

Ulna

Tensegrity and biotensegrity

The sculpture on the left is Kenneth Snelson's *Needle Tower*—a *tensegrity* structure. Its solid rods are held in place by a web of *tensioned* cables. The strength (or int*egrity*) of the whole structure (system) comes from the tension within the cables, rather than the strength of the rods. When this architectural principle is applied to living bodies, it's called *biotensegrity*.

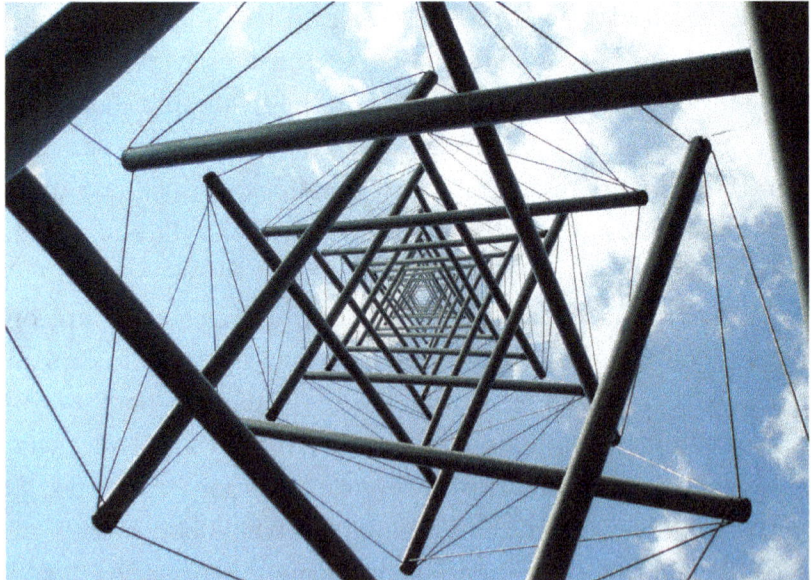

Biotensegrity recognises the body as a naturally integrated, living system, governed more by the laws of nature than classical mechanics. Its symmetry, stability, and responsiveness rely on a moment-by-moment balance of tension and compression forces distributed through the entire structure. Any localised change—a tight hamstring, a broken bone, a surgical mesh implant, or even wearing high heels—can alter the whole system's shape, function, and internal environment.

From this perspective, healing and movement are not just biomechanical responses but coordinated, whole-body adaptations. This approach helps explain why small changes in posture, alignment, or tension can ripple through the system and affect everything from pain and balance to digestion and breathing.

Biotensegrity invites us to think less about fixing individual parts and more about how the whole body works together as a unified, adaptive system. It's a model that aligns closely with fascia-aware practice—and helps make sense of the subtle, interconnected effects that hands-on therapies often reveal.

Both the biomechanical and biotensegrity models provide useful insights, but neither fully explains how the body moves. As a clinician, I found it helpful to combine both models to better understand movement and injury.

"The body is basically a tensegrity structure." —Donald Ingber (1998)

"If the behaviour of living organisms were to follow the laws of classical mechanics, then lifting a heavy weight would cause muscles to tear, discs to rupture, vertebrae to be crushed and blood vessels to burst ..." —Graham Scarr (2002), citing Levin (2002)

The anatomy of perception: a glimpse into physiotherapy education

Helen's life revolves around three passions: her cherished friendships, her teaching job, and her peaceful, Japanese-inspired garden. When she agreed to sit down for an interview as part of my research into anatomy education in New Zealand, I knew I was about to hear from someone with extensive experience, particularly in the world of physiotherapy teaching.

As a senior lecturer in a university health sciences department, Helen has been shaping the future of physiotherapists, occupational therapists, nurses, and other health professionals for over two decades. She teaches Human Anatomy, Physiology, and Kinesiology to first-year students, laying the groundwork for their healthcare training. However, as Helen points out, the anatomy she teaches is framed through a traditional lens—one that divides the body into separate parts like muscles, bones, and organs, each functioning independently.

In the first year of the programme, students learn about the body's key organ systems, including the musculoskeletal, respiratory, and nervous systems. They study these systems by focusing on the structure and function of each part, but there's one problem: fascia, the connective tissue that holds everything together, is barely mentioned. It's briefly touched on during one of their lectures about connective tissue, but little attention is given to it.

Helen explains: "We don't emphasise fascia much. It's only mentioned when it's relevant to the area we're teaching about, like the crural fascia in the leg or the iliotibial tract in the thigh. It's not the star of the show. We focus on the parts our students need to know about."

When students get the chance to observe bodies in the dissection labs, they sometimes glimpse fascia—if it hasn't already been removed. "The embalmed specimens offer a rare opportunity to see fascia in its natural environment—visible, durable, and sometimes surprisingly strong—but they usually don't notice it," she says. "They're always amazed by the iliotibial band. That's when they realise how tough these structures are."

Despite these moments, fascia doesn't leave a lasting impression. "Connective tissue is only briefly mentioned in the introductory lectures. We don't test their knowledge on fascia," Helen admits. "It's just not the focus. The big picture things—like muscles, bones, joints, organs, and nervous system—get all the attention. Fascia gets left behind."

The limited focus on fascia reflects a broader trend in physiotherapy education. The traditional, anatomised musculoskeletal model dominates how students learn about anatomy, physiology, pathology, kinesiology, and treatment methods. While it's useful for teaching basic anatomy to beginners, it overlooks the crucial roles fascia plays in the body.

Helen acknowledges this gap: "It sounds like there's so much more to fascia than we teach. Maybe we're only scratching the surface, and now I'm not sure if what we teach is enough. We're still mainly focused on muscles and bones. Fascia's role in pain, healing, and movement isn't something we dive into deeply."

By the end of our conversation, Helen wondered whether it was time to rethink how fascia is integrated into the curriculum. "I do think there's a lot more to fascia that we could be teaching," she said thoughtfully. "It sounds like fascia's role in pain, healing, and movement can't be ignored for much longer. Maybe it's time for it to be seen as more than an afterthought."

Musculoskeletal medicine and healthcare

Musculoskeletal medicine focuses on preventing, diagnosing, treating, and rehabilitating conditions that affect the body's muscles, bones, joints, and related tissues. Common musculoskeletal disorders—such as back pain, arthritis, sports injuries,

Consider how the traditional focus on the body's musculoskeletal system has influenced the treatment you've received from your healthcare providers. Was it as effective as you'd hoped in supporting your body's health and healing?

and conditions like fibromyalgia or carpal tunnel syndrome—can severely impact quality of life.

Healthcare professionals like physiotherapists, sports physicians, orthopaedic surgeons, and rheumatologists help individuals manage these conditions. They use a mix of physical therapy, exercise, manual therapy, medication, injections, and lifestyle advice to reduce pain, restore function, and improve overall wellbeing.

Flesh and Bones—the Living Wetsuit

05

"Fascia forms an integrating tissue system that unifies the body connecting all parts together. It helps all areas of the body to work together in coordinated patterns of movement. Therefore, the structure and function of each individual part of the body as a whole is to some extent controlled by the fascia. As a result, fascia has an important role in maintaining our health."
—Michael Kern (2001)

We all know that our bodies consist of both soft and hard parts—our flesh and bones. In humans and other animals, "flesh" refers to all the soft, meaty, and fatty tissue that wraps around our bones. It plays a vital role in keeping us alive, helping us move, breathe, digest food, and fight off infections.

But what happens when a body stops living? Without getting too graphic, most people understand that flesh doesn't last long after death. It breaks down quickly—especially in hot climates or when scavengers are around!

Bones, on the other hand, are much tougher. While flesh soon softens and slips away, bones can survive for hundreds—even thousands—of years. Maybe that's why some of our ancestors imagined the body as a kind of "bone house"—a shelter built of sturdy scaffolding. In Early English, phrases like *bone hall*, *bone dwelling* and *bone house* captured this idea. Some even pictured the soul as a silent guardian, tending to its bony home throughout a lifetime.

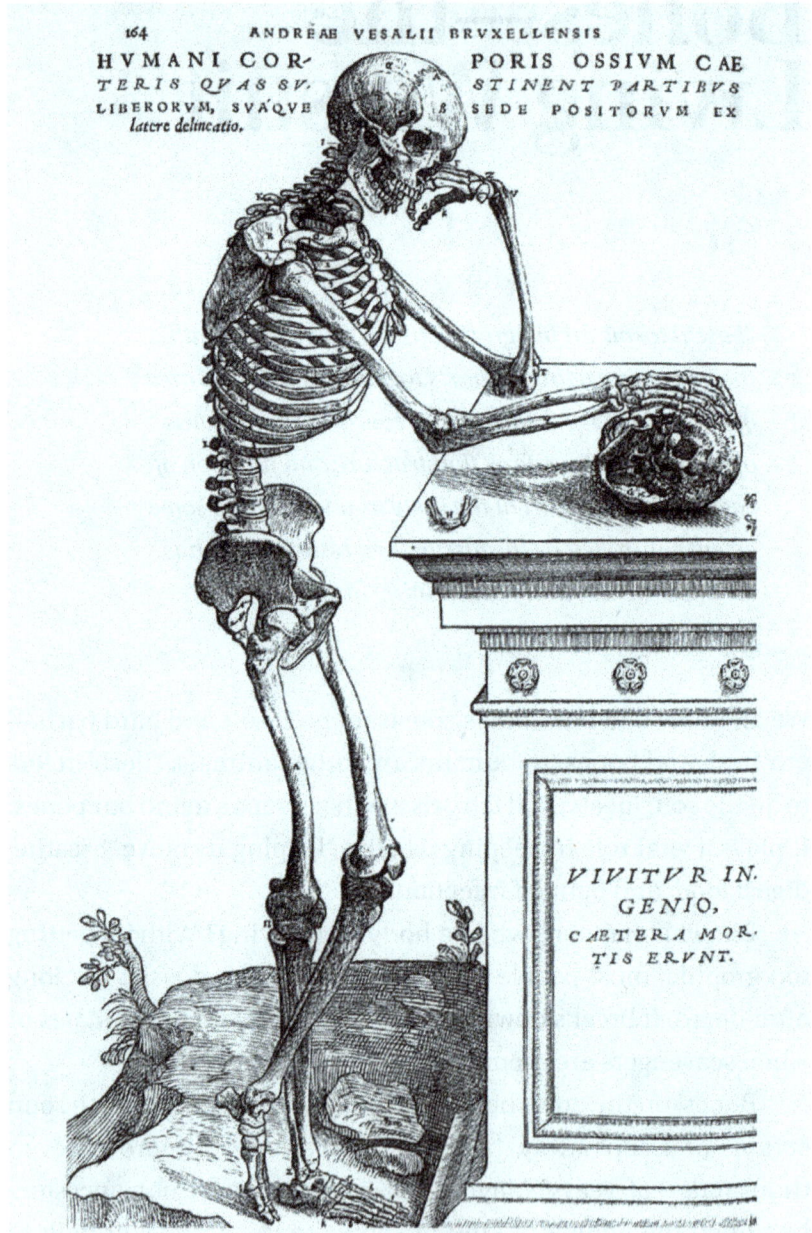

164　　ANDREAE VESALII BRVXELLENSIS
HVMANI COR-　　　　PORIS OSSIVM CAE
TERIS QVAS SV.　　　*STINENT PARTIBVS*
LIBERORVM, SVAQVE　*SEDE POSITORVM EX*
latere delineatio.

*VIVITVR IN-
GENIO,
CAETERA MOR-
TIS ERVNT.*

The Living Wetsuit

Imagine wearing a full-body wetsuit—not the kind you use for surfing or scuba diving, but one that's alive, flexible, and incorporates every part of you. That's the idea behind the "Living Wetsuit" (LWS)—a simple way to grasp how our bodies are naturally whole and alive. Instead of viewing the body as a collection of separate parts, as anatomy books often do, the LWS helps us see it as it truly is—an interconnected whole.

In my last book, I described it as a "living, fleshy, skeleton-hugging body garment ... that surrounds the body's skeleton of bones, and fills up all of the space between them and the body's outer skin surface."

Two key elements make this concept special:

1. **Fascia**—a stretchy, three-dimensional web of tissue that holds everything together. It's what keeps our body parts from being just separate pieces of tissue. No wonder fascia has been called the body's fabric of wholeness (Agneesens, 2001).
2. **Life energy**—the invisible force that makes a body alive rather than an inert structure (discussed in the next chapter).

Without both, we wouldn't have a body—let alone one that moves, grows, and functions as it does.

A living fabric

You can think of it like the canvas in a needlepoint embroidery. In needlepoint, colourful stitches are added onto the fabric to create a design. Similarly, our body's fascia acts as a base fabric, while muscle cells, liver cells, nerves, blood vessels, and even bones are the "stitches" that make up the final form.

A skeleton wearing a "fleshy wetsuit"

The Living Wetsuit (LWS) is a name for the soft and squishy human body-shaped 'garment' of flesh that is worn underneath instead of over the skin. It surrounds the body's skeleton of bones and fills the space between them and the body's outer skin surface. In living people's bodies, the LWS is perfused with and exudes several types of energy—some of which are physically measurable (e.g., electromagnetic energy, heat, sound). The various types of energy collectively form an energy field that envelops the entire body. This energy field normally extends a few centimetres beyond the skin and is visible to some, though not all, people as an aura of pale light.

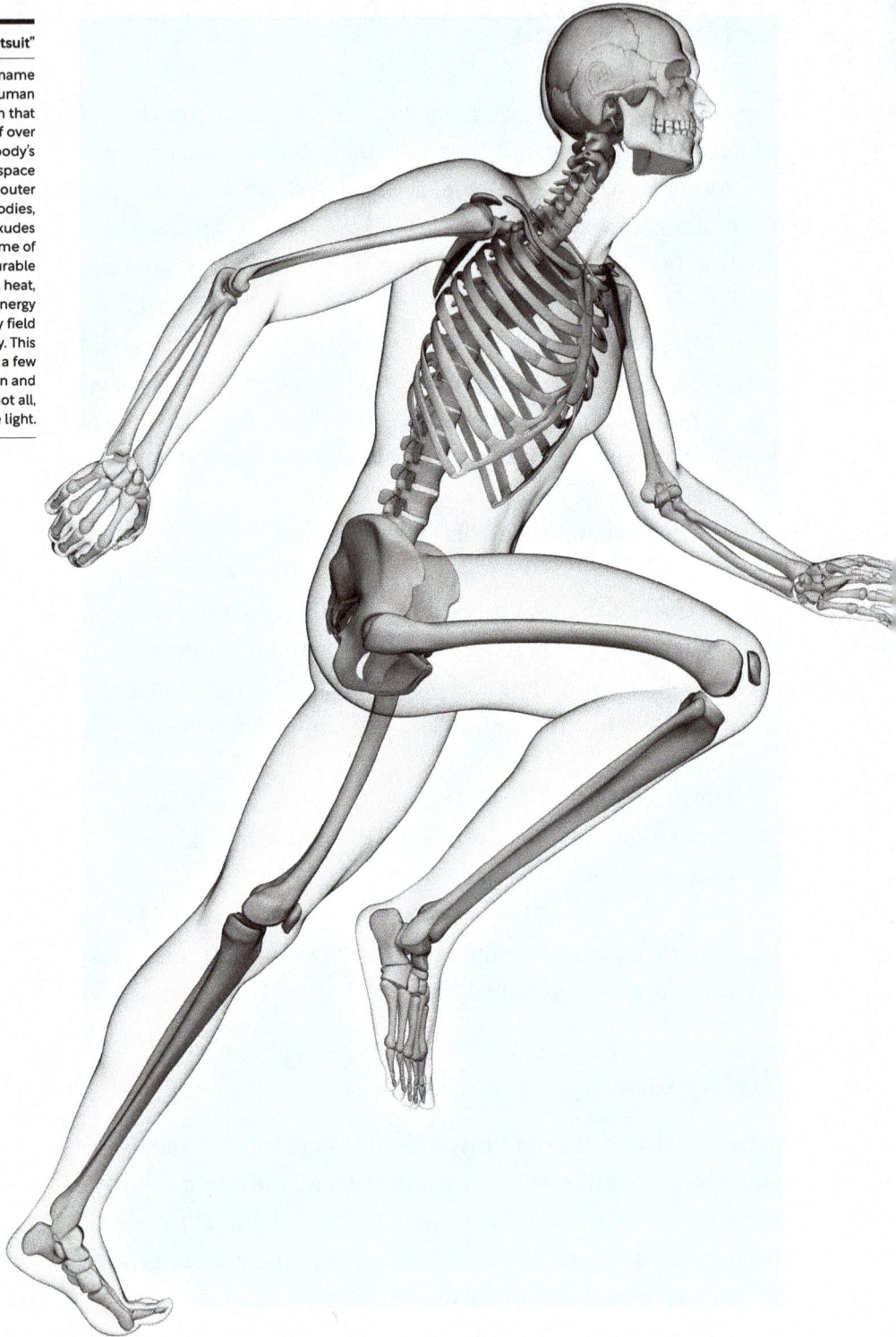

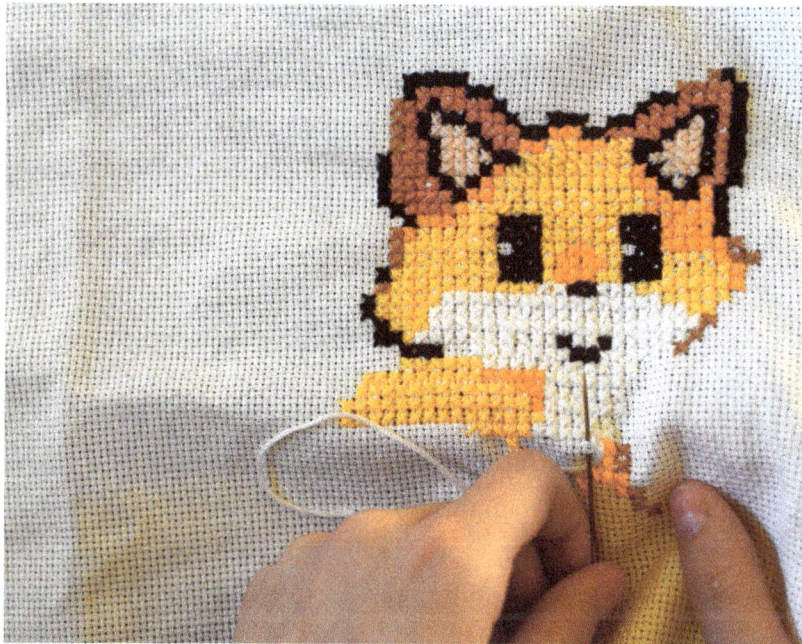

Needlepoint and the body

Needlepoint is a kind of embroidery where yarn is stitched into a canvas following a planned pattern. The finished design gives the picture its shape and purpose. In a similar way, fascia acts like the body's base fabric—with muscles, nerves, blood vessels, and even bones forming the "stitches" that create the body's final form.

Of course, the human body is far more complex than a piece of embroidery. But just like stitches in a needlepoint design, every part of the body relies on the underlying fabric (fascia) to hold it in place. Without it, our body wouldn't be a unified, functioning whole—just a messy heap of biological bits and blobs down on the floor.

Pause for a moment to imagine this: though it's a practical impossibility, if you could leave the fascia intact and remove everything else from the body—bones, nerves, organs, arteries, and veins—you would be left with a kind of three-dimensional blueprint of the body. In essence, a fascial body. It would look something like a huge loofah sponge in the shape of your body.

Now imagine the reverse: if you could remove all the fascia from the body, aside from the bones and a few other structures, you'd be left with a pile of unrecognisable formless stuff (paraphrased from Maitland, 1995).

Myofascia

The word *myofascia* started appearing in medical literature around the mid-20th century as researchers studied a newly identified condition called *myofascial pain syndrome*. The term blends two words:

- *Myo-*, meaning muscle.
- *Fascia*, the connective tissue that surrounds, permeates, and supports muscles.

For a long time, muscles were seen mainly as red contractile tissue that pulls on tendons to move bones. This idea is partly true—but it leaves out fascia, which is equally important. Even today, many health professionals—including physiotherapists, sports doctors, and orthopaedic surgeons—focus mostly on muscles, bones, and joints without fully considering the fascial network that binds and integrates them.

Muscles and fascia: a connected system

Muscles make up about one-third of a person's body weight (Janssen et al., 2000), but they aren't made of muscle cells alone. Fascia surrounds, permeates, and connects every part of our muscles, and also links them with surrounding structures.

Within muscles, fascia:

- **Allows smooth movement**—Fascia lets muscle fibres and bundles glide freely against one another without friction or damage.
- **Distributes force**—It disperses pressure and tension not just through tendons (a type of fascia), but throughout the muscle's interior and surrounding tissues. This allows the

force generated by one contracting muscle to spread across others, helping them work together more efficiently.

- **Provides support**—It houses the vessels and fluid pathways that nourish muscle cells and remove waste.
- **Sends information**—Packed with nerves and sensory nerve endings, fascia plays a vital role in communication between muscles and the rest of the body.

Because of this, muscles and fascia aren't separate—they function as one integrated system. Some experts call them *myofascial units* (Myers, 2014), highlighting the fact that muscles can't function properly without their fascial support.

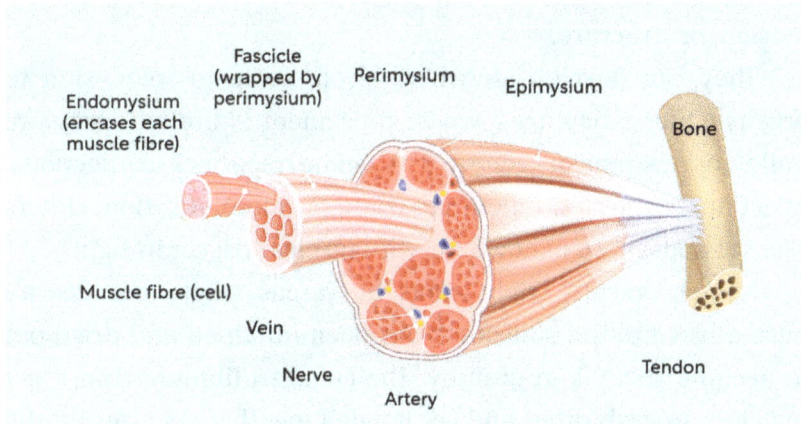

Endomysium (encases each muscle fibre)

Fascicle (wrapped by perimysium)

Perimysium

Epimysium

Bone

Muscle fibre (cell)

Vein

Nerve

Artery

Tendon

Myofascia (muscle + fascia)

A muscle's supporting fascia wraps around three different levels of muscle cells:

(1) the *endomysium*, which covers each individual muscle fibre (or muscle cell),

(2) the *perimysium*, which wraps around each bundle (fascicle) of fibres, and

(3) the *epimysium*, which surrounds the whole muscle.

Despite their different names, these three layers are all part of the same continuous fascial fabric that connects with the rest of the body's fascia.

"There's no such thing as a muscle ... every muscle of the body is surrounded by a smooth fascial sheath, every muscular fascicle is surrounded by fascia, and every fibril is surrounded by fascia ... Therefore, it is the fascia that ultimately determines the length and function of its muscular component ... [The] separation of the fascia and its influence from the muscular component and their influence on each other is imaginary." —John F. Barnes (1990)

Tight spots

A Living Wetsuit (LWS) isn't always in pristine condition. Life happens—not always in ways we would choose—bringing stress, strain, injury, wear, and illness. Some LWSs are born with quirks; others acquire them over time. While resilient and designed to last, they're not invincible.

Tight spots form—areas where the LWS thickens, stiffens, and loses its glide. They may feel sore or tender, but just as often they're silent troublemakers—hidden yet disruptive. Some come with a label: myofascial pain syndrome, plantar fasciitis, or tennis elbow, trigger points, adhesions, or scar tissue. Others remain nameless. But all involve a shift in the fascial fabric—its texture, hydration, tension, or structure.

They can develop anywhere—from scalp to soles, skin to organs. Often, they arise where movement is limited, pressure builds, or repair hasn't gone to plan. Some trace back to infections, injections, surgeries, repetitive strain, or immobilisation. Others seem to appear out of nowhere, with no clear trigger in sight.

Microscopically, tight spots are areas where the fascia's once-gooey ground substance has been inflamed and dried out to become sticky and gummy. The collagen fibres within it get too close to each other and get tangled together. As a result, the fascial tissue sticks where it should glide, clumps where it should flow. It squeezes vessels, chokes nerves, and drags on surrounding structures. Movement gets harder. Pain lingers longer.

Why tight spots matter

Tight spots can become focal points of tension, eventually contributing to the development of local and widespread movement restrictions. The LWS's innate interconnectedness means that a tight spot (a localised area of tissue stuckness) can pull and drag into other areas of its fabric—just like when you grip and pull on a piece of clothing. As time goes by, these pull-strain lines can produce problems far removed from the original area of stuckness.

Just like a snagged thread in a sweater, they pull into the fascial fabric around them and send strain radiating outward—up the leg, across the back, into the neck. A sore shoulder may stem from a tight foot. A lingering headache may trace back to jaw tension. The body adapts, compensates, and eventually protests.

Between them, tight spots and pull-strain lines can pull and twist the LWS, along with the cells, tissues, organs, and systems it contains. Unless remedied, this may distort the shape, position, relative alignment, and functioning of the body's parts. Dense and tense LWS fabric loses elasticity and "give", making it less able to absorb and disperse shock. This raises the risk of further injury and pain—as anyone recovering from surgery or managing a frozen shoulder, ruptured Achilles, or repetitive strain injury can attest.

Tight spots and pull-strain lines can effectively shrink, tether, or twist the LWS, changing the way this fleshy garment fits over the bones. This can compress the joints between them, alter their alignment, and restrict their range of movement. Squashed or stretched soft structures—like glands and organs—may become damaged and unable to function normally. A poorly fitting LWS can squash or abnormally stretch sensitive nerve endings, the spinal cord, or even the brain. This can not only cause pain, but alter how the nervous system senses, processes, and responds to information.

They can also block or redirect the normal circulation of fluids—blood, lymph, interstitial fluid, cerebrospinal fluid—interfering with nourishment, waste removal, immune function, and healing. In some cases, this can contribute to swelling (oedema) in the feet, hands, or face—or more critically, the lungs or brain.

If left untreated, some tight spots will resolve with time, especially if the person is healthy, hydrated, and active. But many hang around and accumulate. The LWS slowly stiffens, loses ease,

Pull-strain lines

Tight spots pull into the surrounding tissue, a bit like a snag pulling through a knitted jumper. These forces can travel through the body's 'living wetsuit' via pull-strain lines, creating trouble far from the original source. Over time, as more tight spots and pull-strain lines develop, the LWS can effectively shrink, twist, or become too tight—disrupting the structures inside it, including bones, joints, nerves, and blood vessels.

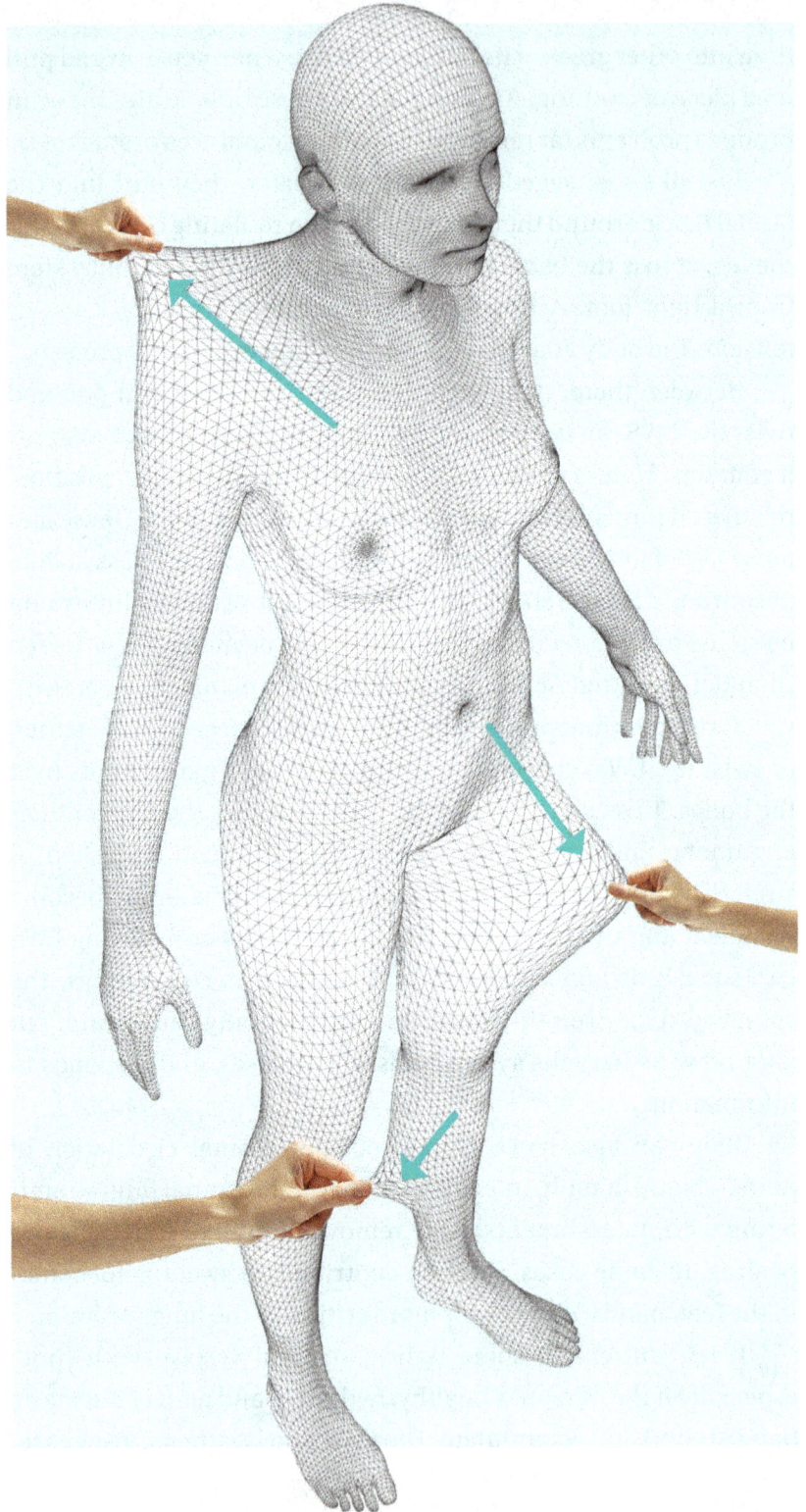

and becomes less forgiving. Before long, it stops moving the way it used to. It doesn't bounce back. It hurts. The body becomes more effortful to live in.

Worse still, the person wearing it (and sometimes their health professionals) may not even realise these tight spots exist. They may not recognise their link to other, more visible health issues—especially the stubborn, complex, or long-lasting ones that haven't responded well to conventional treatment. They may assume this is just ageing, or that nothing can be done. But that isn't true.

With the right attention, tight spots can soften, rehydrate, and release. The LWS remembers its shape and how it should move—and, given the chance, it will return to its healthier natural state.

"Fascial strains can slowly tighten, causing the body to lose its physiologic adaptive capacity. Over time, the tightness spreads like a pull in a sweater ... Flexibility and spontaneity of movement are lost ... setting up the body for more trauma, pain, and limitation of movement." —John F. Barnes (1990)

Myofascial meridians

Many manual and movement therapists are already familiar with tight spots and the pull-strain lines that radiate from them. But these are not the same as *myofascial meridians.*

Pull-strain lines are signs of imbalance—patterns of strain and tension that develop in response to stuckness or dysfunction. Myofascial meridians, on the other hand, are normal anatomical structures—lines of continuity in the body's connective tissue that transmit force, movement, and restriction across distant regions.

The term "myofascial meridians" was coined in the 1990s by Thomas Myers, a Structural Integration practitioner. Myers proposed that the fascia within and between muscles connects them into long, continuous chains of myofascial tissue—*myofascial meridians*. He likened them to railway lines linking distant stations across the body, which led to them also being known as *Anatomy Train lines.*

Dissection and imaging studies have confirmed the existence of these chains, demonstrating that tension in one part of a meridian can indeed affect function elsewhere. These meridians offer a practical map for understanding how structure and function interrelate.

I attended a short Anatomy Trains workshop several years ago, taught by a skilled international instructor named Raymond. He had initially trained in New Zealand as a massage therapist and was soon employed by an international professional dance company. His dancer-patients enjoyed and responded well to his treatments, which enabled them to continue their work with minimum disruption. Raymond, however, became concerned as he noticed the dancers' injuries and pain kept recurring. Seeking to improve on this situation, he researched the matter and then trained as a Structural Integration practitioner, eventually qualifying as a teacher of the *Anatomy Trains* method.

In the workshop, he introduced us to the idea of meridians as functional lines of connection. One of those he specifically taught us about—the superficial back line—extends from the soles of the feet, up the back of the legs and spine, over the skull, and ends at the forehead. A restriction in one area—like tight calves—could contribute to back pain or even headaches. He suggested that stretching the feet might relieve tension in the neck.

This view reframes pain and movement as whole-body phenomena. If one part gets stuck, the entire system adapts around it. Treatment, therefore, isn't just about where it hurts—it's about finding where the fascia isn't moving.

Much of our class time was spent learning two essential skills: body reading and palpation. Body reading meant observing how someone stood and moved to spot areas of imbalance—what Raymond called "the short and long bits"—in the body's structure.

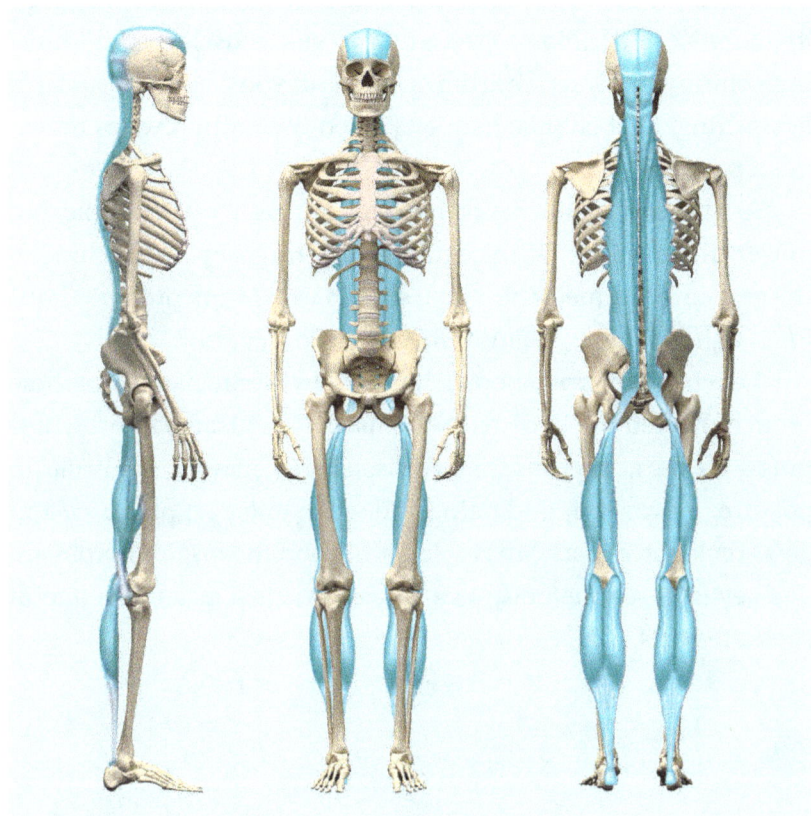

Palpation involved using our hands to feel where the tissues glided smoothly and where they were stuck. "Pain often shows up in one place, but the real problem can be somewhere else," he reminded us. "That's why you have to feel for where the fascia isn't moving."

When it came to treatment, he emphasised the need for precision. "Don't push too hard," he cautioned. "You need to feel which layer you're working on. The goal isn't to stretch muscle—it's to restore glide between the layers of fascia inside and around it."

He also encouraged movement during treatment. "Ask the person to move in the direction that's stuck," he said. "That increases the stretch and makes the treatment more effective."

Yet he was careful not to overstate fascia's role. "Good treatment is never about just one thing," he said. "You might also need to mobilise stiff joints, strengthen weak muscles, and—most importantly—engage the brain. The nervous system controls everything. Real change happens when the brain rewires movement patterns."

At the end of the workshop, he left us with a simple but powerful metaphor: "Think of fascia like the gears of a machine. If the gears are jammed, the whole system won't work properly. Your job is to free them up so movement can flow again."

Leaving the workshop, I had a new appreciation for how interconnected the body truly is. Fascia isn't just a passive wrapping—it's an active, responsive tissue that plays a vital role in posture, movement, and pain. And when one part of the system gets stuck, the effects can ripple far beyond the original problem. The key is to see the body as a whole—not just as a collection of separate parts.

The Mind-Body

06

"Connectivity and unity are organismic truths."
—Agneessens (2001)

Separated or connected?

Think about the difference between a live chicken roaming a farm and a neatly packaged tray of chicken pieces at the supermarket. One is a whole, living creature, scratching at the dirt and clucking away. The other has been cut apart into convenient sections, ready for cooking.

Now, compare your body as you sit here reading this to a body in an anatomy lab—generously donated by its former owner. Yours is alive, complete, and functioning. The other has been carefully dissected for medical study. Both are called "bodies", but they're not the same. Yours is warm, breathing, and moving. The other is lifeless, cold, and stiff. One is whole. The other has been taken apart.

This is where things get tricky. Without really thinking about it, society—especially in science and medicine—has blurred the line between living bodies and the ones described in anatomy textbooks. We've been taught to picture our bodies as a collection of separate parts, like an anatomical diagram or a list of organs. But living bodies don't work like that. They aren't just stitched-together pieces; they are dynamic, connected systems.

In reality, living bodies are more than just their physical structures. They include fascia—an interconnected web of tissue that holds everything together. They contain energies, signals, and other subtle but vital connections that don't show up in anatomy textbooks. If we truly want to understand health and healthcare, we need to think beyond the conventional, dissected view of the body. The anatomical perspective is useful, but it's also limited. And those limits shape how we think about health and medicine.

In the next few chapters, we'll explore the more subtle, often-overlooked aspects of the human body—things that aren't easily captured in a photograph but are essential to understanding what it really means to be alive.

What do we mean by "body"?

Different definitions highlight different aspects of what a body is:

- A tangible, physical form.
- A person's mortal form, distinct from their soul or consciousness.
- A lifeless body (a corpse or cadaver).
- A collection of organs, tissues, cells, and molecules that make up a physical human body.
- The main parts of a person's body, as opposed to its seemingly less significant ones.
- A physically whole body that functions as an organised unit.
- A biological structure that influences—and is influenced by—more than its physical form.
- A person.

Which of these definitions fits best? Or is a living body something more than any one of them can capture?

Dr. Still and the wholeness of the body

Andrew Taylor Still (1828–1917) was a self-taught frontier doctor who viewed the body quite differently from most medical professionals of his era. While many of them learned about bodies by dissecting cadavers in big city medical schools, Dr. Still also drew on hands-on experience, keen observation, and his own research.

In his day, mainstream medicine often involved harsh treatments like bloodletting, purging, and toxic drugs—methods that were not only painful but sometimes deadly. After losing three of his four children to meningitis, Dr Still became determined to find a better way. His search led him to develop osteopathy, a medical approach that focused on supporting the body's ability to heal itself—if given the right conditions.

One of Dr. Still's biggest insights concerned how we think about the body. He argued that breaking the body into separate parts—like chopping a chicken into drumsticks, wings, and breasts—misses something vital. A chicken is only a chicken when all its parts are present and working together. The same is true for people. He believed that studying anatomy shouldn't just focus on isolated pieces but *also* the living connections that bring them together as a whole.

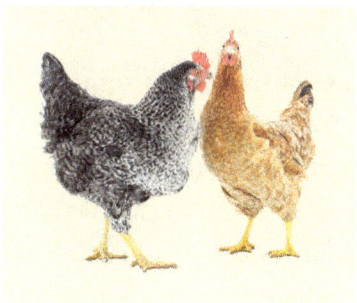

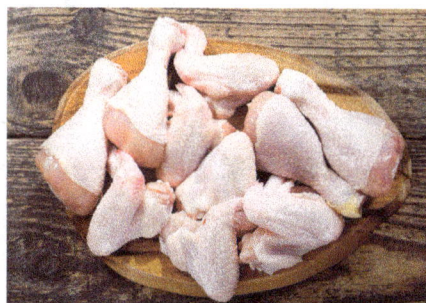

Whole and alive hens and dissected dead chicken pieces

Dr. Still saw fascia as a crucial part of this wholeness. He described it as the unifying tissue that holds everything together and plays a role in health from birth to death. He even suggested that understanding fascia could reveal more about how the body works than studying any other part. In his words, fascia is "universal in man and equal in self to all other parts". He believed that truly grasping its role could bring "more rich golden thought" than any other area of anatomy.

So, if we really want to understand the body, we need to consider *both* perspectives: the individual parts and how they all come together as a living whole.

Beyond the physical

For centuries, anatomists have studied the human body using their physical senses—primarily sight and touch. They've carefully dissected, examined, and mapped out every muscle, bone, and organ. In earlier times, some even relied on smell, taste, and hearing to gather information (though tasting tissue is thankfully no longer part of modern anatomy!).

This approach has given us incredible knowledge about the body's structure. We've learned a great deal by viewing it as a physical object—something we can see, touch, and measure. But here's the catch: while this method works well for understanding body parts, it falls short when it comes to understanding what makes a body alive.

A living body isn't just a collection of parts—it's something more. Movement, energy, awareness, the ability to think and heal all go beyond what can be fully explained by dissecting tissue or analysing biological structures. Even with the most advanced scientific tools, the essence of life itself remains something we struggle to measure or define. Yet, whatever that "something more" is, it's real—just because we can't put it under a microscope doesn't mean it doesn't exist.

By focusing only on the physical, we risk missing the bigger picture. A body on an anatomy table and a body walking, breathing, and experiencing the world may have the same physical components, but one is just a shell, while the other is *alive*.

More than just science

Throughout history, philosophers, healers, artists, and scholars from all walks of life have studied the human form and function—each bringing their own unique perspectives. Some have examined the body through ancient wisdom, intuition, or lived experience. Others have mapped it through movement, energy, or even language.

But in the past 500 years—a blink in the grand timeline of human history—our fascination with science has overshadowed these other ways of knowing. The rise of scientific thinking has led to incredible discoveries, but it has also come at a cost—the dismissal, or even outright rejection, of other valuable ways of knowing. If something can't be weighed, measured, photographed, or written into an equation, it's often brushed aside.

This book challenges that mindset. It refuses to limit our understanding of the body to just one narrow lens. Instead, it invites us to explore all the ways we can make sense of our living, breathing selves—whether through science, philosophy, history, or perspectives that don't fit neatly into a lab report.

If we accept that wholeness is rooted in connection, then we must ask: "What exactly are we connected to?" Our bodies are not isolated biological systems. They are deeply intertwined with our thoughts, emotions, and broader cultural understandings of bodies and health.

This chapter explores the first of two holistic health models: the mind-body approach and Te Whare Whā (discussed in the next chapter)—that recognise and integrate these connections in healthcare.

Mind and body: a powerful connection

We often think of the mind and body as separate, but in reality, they're deeply connected. The way we think, feel, and behave affects our physical health—and vice versa. This idea is known as the mind-body (or body-mind) connection.

Rather than being two separate things, the mind and the body form one integrated system. Sure, we can talk about them separately—like two sides of the same coin—but in a living, breathing person, they constantly influence each other. Your thoughts and emotions impact your body's health, just as physical experiences shape your mental state. For example, positive thoughts can trigger the release of feel-good chemicals like serotonin and dopamine, while stress can cause muscle tension or even make you feel sick.

But where exactly does the mind come from? That's a question people have debated for centuries. Some believe the mind resides in the brain, heart, or gut, while others think it is something more abstract—connected to the soul or consciousness. Ancient thinkers like Aristotle believed intelligence was housed in the heart, while Herophilus argued it was in the brain. Even today, scientists and philosophers continue to explore this mystery.

The four minds

Some researchers suggest we actually have four different types of minds, each connected to different parts of our body and brain:

1. Soul-mind—linked to deeper awareness or spirituality.
2. Reptilian mind (body-mind)—responsible for our most basic survival instincts, like fight-or-flight reactions.
3. Limbic mind (emotional mind)—processes emotions and social connections.
4. Neocortex (rational mind)—controls logic, problem-solving, and reasoning.

Each of these plays a role in shaping our thoughts, emotions, and overall health.

What is psychology?

The study of the mind (psyche) and behaviour is called psychology. It explores how we think, feel, and act—both consciously and unconsciously. Psychologists and psychiatrists—notice the "psych" in their titles—work to understand and treat mental health conditions using methods like talk therapy, medication, and other techniques. Some therapies focus on talking through emotions, while others, like cognitive behavioural therapy (CBT) or meditation, help people rewire thought patterns to improve well-being.

Mind-body practices: science meets wellness

"Healthcare's worst-kept secret: Treat the mind to improve physical health." —Eric Arzubi

Even the National Cancer Institute, a leading medical research organisation in the United States, recognises that mind-body (and body-mind) practices can improve health. These include:

- Meditation and mindfulness—calming the mind to reduce stress.
- Yoga and tai chi—combining movement with breath control.
- Hypnosis and guided imagery—using focused thought to influence the body.
- Art and music therapy—expressing emotions creatively.
- Laughter yoga and massage—releasing tension and boosting mood.

Some of these could also be seen as treating the body to benefit the mind. Others include breathwork and Eye Movement Desensitisation and Reprocessing (EDMR), a technique used in trauma therapy.

Whatever we call them, these techniques show that the mind isn't just a passive observer—it actively shapes our health and well-being. Science is finally catching up to what ancient traditions have long understood: the mind and body are inseparably connected, and it's important to take care of them both.

A founder's journey from burnout to holistic wellbeing

Nick didn't set out to create a workplace wellbeing platform. He wasn't chasing inspiration—he was recovering from exhaustion.

In his late twenties, Nick was pouring everything he had into a previous startup. The long hours, relentless pressure, and weight of responsibility eventually caught up with him. His body gave out, and he ended up in hospital—burned out, run-down, and completely depleted. It was a wake-up call he couldn't ignore.

Recovery wasn't quick, and it certainly wasn't easy. It took years—and a fundamental rethinking of how he approached life. Nick began working with a psychotherapist, a personal trainer, and a nutritionist. Slowly, he started to rebuild. But something deeper shifted, too. He came to understand that wellbeing isn't just about food, or fitness, or mental health—it's about how those things interact. He saw firsthand that the mind affects the body, and the body affects the mind. Healing, he realised, has to work in both directions.

That insight became the foundation for the platform Nick eventually launched in 2024. Built around the understanding that mental and physical wellbeing are inseparable—and mutually reinforcing—it offers a flexible, person-centred approach to self-care. The concept is simple but powerful: employers provide staff with a wellbeing allowance, which can be used as digital tokens in a carefully curated marketplace.

Whether someone is looking to calm their nervous system through counselling or mindfulness (mind-to-body), or to improve mood and resilience through massage, yoga, or physiotherapy (body-to-mind), the platform meets them there. Employees can choose what they actually need—dental care, nutritional advice, coaching, movement therapies, and more.

It's not a one-size-fits-all solution. It's a consciously designed system that recognises the complexity of real people—and gives them the freedom to care for themselves in ways that work for *them*. Not a prescription. Not a programme. Just the space, and the support, to come back to themselves.

The early results speak for themselves. Since its launch, the platform has expanded internationally and received glowing feedback. Users have reported a 30% improvement in their overall wellbeing, with noticeable increases in workplace engagement and retention. For many, this is the first time they've truly had the freedom and support to care for their wellbeing on their terms.

Nick built the platform so others wouldn't have to hit rock bottom to realise how important their health is. His journey from burnout to balance has become a bridge—helping others move beyond surface-level wellness perks and toward something deeper, more lasting, and more human.

One mind, one body, one step at a time.

Health, Wholeness, and Te Whare Tapa Whā

07

Health and wholeness

In today's Western medical model, health is often seen as the body working the way it should—like a well-oiled machine. If all the physical nuts and bolts are in place, free of disease, and running smoothly, then you're considered healthy. This view focuses on measurable factors like MRI scans, blood pressure readings, blood tests, and fitness levels.

But wellbeing is something bigger. It's not just about your physical body—it includes your mind, emotions, and how connected you feel to others. You could be physically fit but still feel stressed, lonely, or overwhelmed—meaning your wellbeing might still be out of balance.

A simple way to think about it? Imagine a car. Health is making sure the engine runs well, the tyres are pumped, and there's fuel in the tank. Wellbeing is about enjoying the ride—having a sense of purpose, feeling good about where you're headed, and having great company along the way. To truly thrive, we need both.

For many people, though, separating health and wellbeing doesn't feel quite right. They see these as deeply connected—two parts of the same whole.

In fact, the word "health" comes from an Old English root meaning "whole" or "unbroken". This reminds us that true health is about more than the absence of disease and avoiding illness—it's about balance, vitality, and connection. It's a dynamic state, where the body, mind, and environment work together in harmony.

This idea aligns with modern holistic health models, like Te Whare Tapa Whā, in which health is deeply connected to relationships and wholeness. The mind-body model helps balance the relationship between a person's body and mind. Te Whare Tapa Whā expands on this idea, linking physical health to at least three other dimensions of wellbeing. This model recognises the natural connections between physical, mental, social, and spiritual health, as well as a person's relationship with the land and their sense of belonging.

Te Whare Tapa Whā—a holistic approach to health

In 1984, Māori health advocate Sir Mason Durie developed the Te Whare Tapa Whā model in response to the health challenges faced by Māori communities in New Zealand (Aotearoa), especially the structural inequities and barriers within the Western healthcare system.

The need for a new model
In the late 1970s, research by the Māori Women's Welfare League brought attention to significant health disparities between Māori and European New Zealanders, particularly in mental health. Māori—especially young people—were found to have higher rates of anxiety, mood disorders, substance abuse, and suicidal

thoughts than non-Māori. These findings highlighted the Western medical system's failure to effectively meet the needs of Māori communities.

As a psychiatrist, Durie saw firsthand the limitations of a narrow, symptom-focused approach. Treating only the visible signs of illness wasn't enough. He believed that health (*hauora*) was more than just the absence of disease; it was about overall wellbeing.

A meeting house of health

Te Whare Tapa Whā is inspired by the Māori meeting house (*wharenui*), which has four walls. Each wall represents a key dimension of health:

1. *Taha tinana* (physical health)—The condition and function of the body.
2. *Taha hinengaro* (mental health)—Thoughts, emotions, and psychological wellbeing.
3. *Taha whānau* (family and social health)—Relationships with family, friends, and community.
4. *Taha wairua* (spiritual health)—A sense of connection to the wider world, including culture, ancestors, and personal spiritual beliefs.

Te Whare Tapa Whā

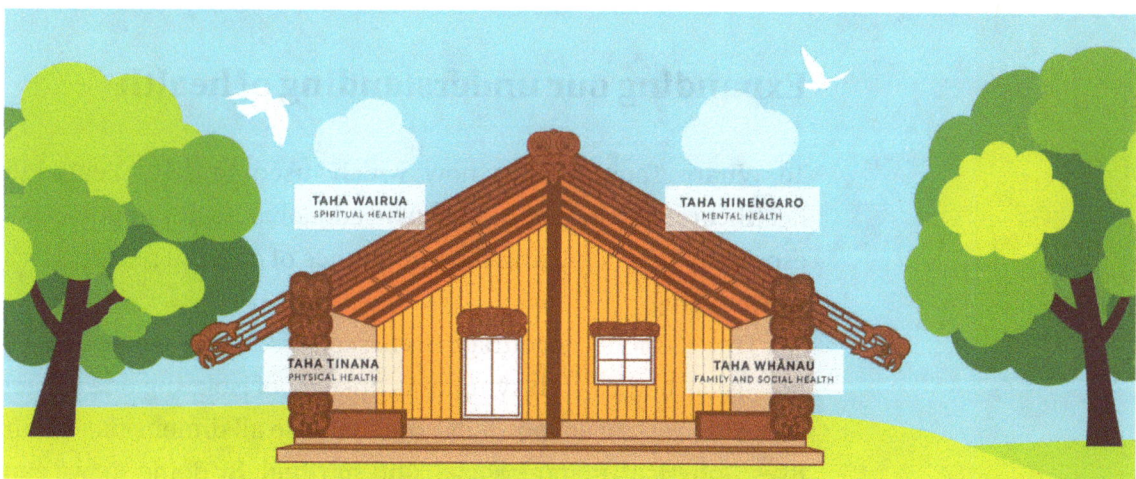

Just as a meetinghouse cannot stand without four walls, a person's wellbeing depends on each of these dimensions. Each wall supports the others, just as the house itself is supported by the land on which it stands. If one is weak or damaged, the whole structure—a person's health and wellbeing—is affected. When seen this way, it is clear that our health is shaped not just by individual choices but by our relationships, our communities, and also the land we live on.

A revolutionary idea

In the 1980s, many New Zealand doctors viewed health through a biomedical lens, focusing on the body's physical symptoms. The idea that mental, social, and spiritual factors played a key role in health was considered radical. But Durie believed that true health was about nurturing the whole person, not just treating symptoms.

One of the most debated aspects of Te Whare Tapa Whā was its emphasis on spirituality. Western medicine often overlooked spiritual wellbeing, yet for many Māori, spirituality was deeply linked to their cultural practices, language (*te reo*), and the natural world. Durie's model challenged traditional healthcare and encouraged a broader view of what a person's body is and what it means for it to be healthy.

Expanding our understanding of health

Te Whare Tapa Whā is now widely used in New Zealand's healthcare system and has influenced global health approaches, especially in recognising the importance of cultural perspectives on wellbeing.

Durie's model encourages us to see ourselves as whole beings, not just as bodies with symptoms. Instead of isolating one aspect of health, we can acknowledge and balance all dimensions of our lives—physical, mental, social, and spiritual. By doing so, we can make more informed, compassionate decisions about how to care for ourselves and others.

True health is not just about being symptom-free—it's about being well in every sense of the word. Whether through our physical health, mental wellbeing, social connections, or spiritual awareness, we are always striving for a state of dynamic wholeness, where all parts of our lives are in balance and functioning optimally.

This holistic understanding of health has also shaped policy and practice in New Zealand, particularly in areas where cultural perspectives on wellbeing have historically been overlooked. One example is New Zealand's Accident Compensation Corporation (ACC), which has changed over time to embrace a more inclusive approach—one that acknowledges the importance of cultural safety in healthcare.

ACC and cultural safety: a new approach to fairer healthcare

The ACC is a government-owned national accident insurance scheme established in 1974 to prevent the health and legal systems from being overwhelmed by accident-related lawsuits. The idea was simple: accidents happen, people get hurt, and instead of blaming individuals, the whole community takes responsibility for their care—in exchange for the right to sue for damages.

I first learned about this major shift in the New Zealand healthcare environment at my physiotherapy cohorts' graduation ceremony. The guest speaker, an orthopaedic surgery professor who'd recently immigrated from South Africa, spoke with knowledge and enthusiasm about what he saw as a groundbreaking step forward in medical care. His perspective made me appreciate just how unique and progressive New Zealand's approach to accident compensation now was compared to other countries' systems where legal battles over injuries were common.

Over time, the ACC has evolved, and in 2024, it introduced

Kawa Whakaruruhau—a newly updated cultural safety policy aimed at making sure that their Māori clients (kiritaki) and their extended families (whānau) feel welcomed, respected, and receive care that leads to much-needed improvement in their health outcomes.

For years, Māori have faced barriers to accessing care that is meaningful and culturally appropriate to them—barriers that have contributed to slower recovery and poorer health outcomes. The ACC's updated approach now makes cultural safety a core part of the care it funds. All ACC-affiliated service providers—including acupuncturists, doctors, physiotherapists, clinic receptionists, and other healthcare staff—are now required to complete cultural safety training. While the primary aim is to improve care for Māori New Zealanders, the policy is designed to benefit all patients by fostering a more respectful, inclusive, and effective healthcare system.

To help put these principles into practice, the ACC recommends three simple but powerful steps for providers:

1. Recognise your own biases—Everyone holds unconscious beliefs that can affect how they treat others. The first step is becoming aware them.
2. Reflect on cultural safety practices—The ACC offers tools to help providers assess how they interact with people from different cultural backgrounds.
3. Engage in conversations with colleagues—Open, ongoing discussions about cultural safety help build awareness and drive meaningful change across the healthcare system.

However, policies alone don't create change, and people don't always follow recommendations. That's why professional registration bodies—like the New Zealand Physiotherapy Board and the Medical Council of New Zealand—play a critical role in making these principles become part of everyday healthcare practice. They do this through ongoing professional development (CPD) requirements, educational resources, and formal monitoring to ensure cultural safety remains a priority in patient care.

The ACC further reinforces these efforts through clinic accreditation processes, adding another layer of accountability. These processes go beyond simply checking whether the providers, whose services they're funding, deliver effective physical treatments—they also assess whether clinics actively create an environment where all patients feel heard, respected, and understand their care. These regular reviews help the ACC uphold cultural safety as more than just a policy on paper—ensuring it remains an active, ongoing commitment in New Zealand's diverse healthcare system.

At the time, while still practising as a physiotherapist, this meant deepening my understanding of both the ACC's and my profession's cultural safety requirements. I did this by studying the ACC's and the physiotherapy profession's criteria on their websites, reading their cultural safety policies and continuing professional education requirement documents, attending online and in-person cultural safety seminars, and engaging in work-place discussions on the topic.

More importantly, it meant being consistently aware of my patients' identities, individual circumstances, and culture-specific needs—and applying this awareness to my practice. A key part of this was writing and submitting at least one reflective statement on cultural safety each year. This wasn't just a box-ticking exercise—it required me to think deeply about cultural safety in real-world healthcare settings before putting those reflections into words.

The ACC's commitment to cultural safety is part of a broader shift in New Zealand's national healthcare system. It acknowledges that good healthcare isn't just about treating injuries—it's about ensuring that every patient, no matter their background,

How does the interconnectedness of the body's physical, mental, social, and spiritual dimensions affect your overall wellbeing, and in what ways can you take more active steps to balance and nurture all four aspects in your own life?

feels valued and supported, and gets treatment that's right for them. Most importantly, it promises that their clients' treatment is physically effective, and above all, achieves results that are fair to everyone, whatever their cultural identity.

These ideas invite us to pause and consider how they might apply in our own lives.

The Quantifiable Energy Body

08

"Everything is energy and that's all there is to it."
—Albert Einstein

Western science tends to focus on what can be seen, touched, and measured. Through this lens, the human body has generally been understood as a solid physical structure—dissected, analysed, and compared to a complex machine. This perspective has shaped modern medicine, grounding it in material evidence and quantifiable data.

But is that the whole story?

It doesn't quite capture the essence of bodies like yours and mine—whole, dynamic, and full of life. In other words, *alive and kicking!*

Energy—more than meets the eye

Anatomy textbooks describe the human body as a structured continuum, from tiny molecules and cells to larger tissues, organs, and organ systems. But if we zoom in further—down to the quantum level—the line between matter and energy begins to blur. Physicists have shown that everything we perceive as solid, including our bodies, is actually made up of vibrating particles and pulsing energy waves.

At the other end of the spectrum, subtle energy fields surround and flow around and through us—though modern science is only beginning to explore these. Ancient cultures, on the other hand, have been working with them for thousands of years. Healers, mystics, and scholars have long recognised that life extends beyond the purely physical. Their insights form the foundation of the next chapter.

Energy is a universal concept, but there are many ways to describe and understand it. It's a bit like the classic story of the blind scholars and the elephant—each one feels a different part and believes they know the whole. No single viewpoint captures the full picture. The goal here isn't to master every explanation but to open the door to new ways of thinking. Let's keep it simple—and explore together.

Two kinds of body energy

Everything in and around us is made of energy. Every quantum particle, atom, molecule, cell, tissue, and organ is alive with movement. This motion generates electrical impulses and emits electromagnetic fields—some we can measure, while others still lie beyond the reach of today's scientific instruments.

For our purposes, we can think of body energy in two basic forms:

1. **Measurable energy**—Detectable forms of physical energy produced by living systems. This includes electrical, thermal, and electromagnetic activity. (*The focus of this chapter.*)
2. **Subtle energy**—Energies believed to exist at frequencies beyond the reach of current scientific instruments, but long recognised in many spiritual and healing traditions. These are said to animate and influence the body in profound ways. (*The focus of the next chapter.*)

The science of energy in the body

In physics, energy is what makes things move or change. It can also be described as invisible vibrations that carry information and interact with everything around them.

ENERGY TYPE	DESCRIPTION
Kinetic energy	Energy of motion
Potential energy	Stored energy
Thermal energy	Heat produced by metabolism
Sound energy	Vibrations traveling through tissues
Chemical energy	Energy stored in molecular bonds
Electrical energy	Flow of charged particles in nerves and tissues
Magnetic energy	Interaction of electrical currents and magnetic fields
Radiant energy	Emission of light, including biophotons
Mechanical energy	Energy used in movement and muscle function
Solar energy	Absorbed from sunlight; influences vitamin D synthesis

Researchers have made several key discoveries about energy in the human body:

1. Living things emit weak electromagnetic signals.
2. These signals can be detected with sensitive instruments.
3. Our bodies are sensitive to those same signals.
4. Some healers claim to use this energy to promote healing.

Electromagnetic energy in the body—a symphony of forces

Our bodies generate and respond to many forms of energy, with each biological process playing a role—like instruments in an orchestra, each contributing to a harmonious whole. At the heart of this symphony is **electromagnetic energy**, produced by the movement of charged particles. It plays a vital role in communication, regulation, and healing.

Here are some key ways the body generates and uses energy:

- **Piezoelectric energy**—When fascia and bone are stretched or compressed, they produce tiny electrical charges, helping tissues adapt to mechanical forces.
- **Chemical energy**—Stored in molecular bonds and released during biological reactions, powering cells and nerve impulses.
- **Streaming potentials**—Electrical currents created by fluid moving through tissues, influencing cellular behaviour.
- **Thermal radiation**—Every movement and metabolic process generates heat, helping maintain cellular activity and body temperature.
- **Sound waves**—Subtle vibrations generated by movement and metabolism travel through tissue, supporting cell communication.
- **Biophotons**—Cells emit tiny flashes of light, which may support subtle signalling between tissues.
- **Electrical currents**—Crucial for nerve signalling and muscle movement.
- **Magnetic fields**—Generated by these electrical currents, influencing physiological processes.

Energy transmission in the body

The body's physical energies don't stay in one place—they flow, interact, and infuse every part of our system. Some of the most well-known transmission pathways include:

- **Nerves**—Carry electrical signals at speeds up to 120 metres per second (m/sec), enabling rapid communication between the brain and body.
- **Blood, lymph, and interstitial fluid**—Transport nutrients, waste, and energy-rich signals via the body's fluid systems.
- **Cerebrospinal and glymphatic fluid**—Support brain function, detoxification, and neural health.

Fluids are highly efficient energy conductors due to their high conductivity. For example:

- Sound travels at about 1,500 m/sec in water, much faster than through air.
- Light moves at roughly 225 million m/sec in water, and just a bit slower in dense tissues like muscle or bone.
- Electrical signals via nerves travel up to 120 m/sec—fast, but still far slower than signals that may move through the body's fluid-based systems.

Fascia—the body's web of connective tissue—is rich in fluid. It contains hydrated ground substance, interstitial fluid, and vessels that carry lymph and blood. Thanks to this, fascia can act as a high-speed communication network, helping mechanical, electrical, chemical, and possibly even light-based signals travel quickly and efficiently throughout the body.

Fascia as the body's broadband network

Think of fascia as your body's internal broadband system.

Just like a high-speed fibre-optic network connects devices in your home, fascia links every part of you—from head to toe, inside and out. It's not just scaffolding that holds things together—it's a transmission network that moves signals, sensations, nutrients, and information at incredible speed.

Its fluid-rich matrix—filled with structured water, interstitial fluids, lymph, and more—that works a bit like a highly conductive cable. Light, pressure, vibration, electrical signals, and biochemical cues can travel swiftly through this medium, connecting cells, tissues, and systems far faster than nerve impulses alone.

If nerves are like old copper wires (still useful, but slower), fascia is like fibre broadband—fast, multidirectional, and built for flow. And just as good Wi-Fi keeps your devices connected and responsive, well-hydrated, mobile fascia keeps your body communicating clearly, sensing efficiently, and functioning at its best.

When the network's flowing, everything hums. But if fascia becomes dry, stiff, or tangled—like a frayed or overloaded cable—communication slows, glitches appear, and systems start to struggle. That's why fascia-focused self-care and treatment practices like hydration, hands-on and vibration therapies, and even breathwork are so powerful: they help "reboot the system" and keep your body online.

The human biofield

Have you ever felt warmth from someone's hands without them touching you? Or stepped into a room and immediately sensed a "vibe"? These experiences may relate to what many call the **biofield**—a measurable energy field that surrounds and interpenetrates all living things.

The human biofield is a dynamic field generated by the body's cells, tissues, and organs. Think of it like a flowing river system, where countless streams of information merge into a larger current. Many believe that patterns within this field influence physical, emotional, mental, and even spiritual wellbeing.

While science hasn't agreed on a single definition, biofield research has grown in recent decades. Standard medical instruments like electrocardiograms (ECGs) and electroencephalograms (EEGs) already measure the heart's and brain's electrical activity of these organs. Newer technologies—like magnetocardiography (MCG) and magnetoencephalography (MEG)—can now detect their magnetic fields. These pass through tissue more easily than electrical signals, so provide deeper insights into heart and brain function.

In 1998, the National Center for Complementary and Alternative Medicine (NCCAM) was established in the US to explore healing methods that fall outside conventional medicine. Some of this research, including studies at the University of Arizona, focused on the human biofield. Could it be measured, and could therapies like Reiki or Therapeutic Touch influence it? The results suggested the answer to both questions was "yes."

Scientific instruments have confirmed that parts of the biofield—especially electromagnetic emissions—can be detected from a few centimetres to over a metre away from the skin, depending on energy type and instruments used. These findings reinforce the idea that the biofield is a tangible, measurable phenomenon.

Biofield medicine

Healing traditions across the world have long worked with different forms of energy—heat, light, sound, electricity, vibration, and even touch. During my undergraduate physiotherapy (physical therapy) training, substantial parts of the curriculum focused on physiotherapeutic modalities using physical energy. At the time, these were understood primarily in terms of their physiological effects rather than their energetic dimensions.

Many of these techniques have since been removed from

modern physiotherapy programmes, as the profession now focuses more on musculoskeletal and exercise-based therapy. Still, their energy-based principles remain valid.

THERAPY	DEFINITION	THERAPEUTIC EFFECTS
Massage	Hands-on soft tissue manipulation (e.g., percussion, vibration)	Improves circulation, reduces tension, supports lymph flow, promotes relaxation
Hydrotherapy	Use of water in various temperatures (e.g., cold packs, ice baths, hot packs, contrast baths)	Reduces pain and inflammation, aids recovery, supports circulation
Paraffin wax therapy	Heated wax applied to joints or skin	Provides deep heat, relieves stiffness (especially in arthritis)
Infrared radiation	Use of infrared light for tissue heating	Promotes healing and pain relief
Ultraviolet radiation	UV light for therapeutic purposes	Aids skin health, stimulates vitaminD production, has antibacterial properties
Ultrasound therapy	High-frequency sound waves penetrating tissues	Reduces pain and swelling, stimulates repair
Galvanic current	Steady direct current	Enhances circulation and tissue healing
Faradic stimulation	Interrupted current to stimulate muscle contraction	Prevents atrophy, strengthens weak muscles
Iontophoresis	Electrical delivery of medication through skin	Delivers anti-inflammatory or pain-relief drugs locally
Shortwave diathermy	High-frequency electromagnetic heating	Relieves deep tissue pain, increases flexibility
Microwave diathermy	Microwave energy to heat deep tissues	Improves mobility and circulation
Interferential therapy	Overlapping currents to stimulate deep tissues.	Reduces pain, improves blood flow, relaxes muscles
TENS (transcutaneous electrical nerve stimulation)	Low-voltage electrical current via skin pads	Alleviates pain by blocking nerve signals, triggering endorphins

Physical energy-based therapies once taught in physiotherapy

While many of these techniques have fallen out of favour in physiotherapy, new forms of biofield medicine are gaining traction. For example:

- Electrical stimulation is still widely used to promote healing.
- High-Intensity Focused Ultrasound (HIFU) is now used in cancer and tissue therapies.
- Transcranial Magnetic Stimulation (TMS) helps modulate brain function.
- Pulsed Electromagnetic Field (PEMF) therapy is used for pain and wound care.

As science develops more sensitive instruments, our ability to measure and understand the body's subtle electromagnetic activity continues to expand. These tools reconnect traditional healing wisdom with modern technologies, potentially reshaping the future of healthcare.

Healing through vibration

Healing begins with movement—specifically, the subtle vibrations that make up everything in the universe. These vibrations are defined by two key properties: *frequency*, or how fast something oscillates, and *amplitude*, or how intense the vibration is. Every living thing, from individual cells to bodies to entire ecosystems, has its own natural frequency and amplitude.

When these vibrations are in harmony, we feel well. When they're disrupted—by injury, stress, toxins, or emotional strain—imbalance can result, sometimes leading to illness.

External vibrations can also affect us. Some researchers suggest that certain environmental frequencies, whether from technology or other sources, can negatively affect our health. On the other hand, targeted vibrations can help restore harmony to the body's natural rhythms.

This is the basis of vibrational medicine—the idea that applying specific frequencies can support the body's ability to self-regulate and heal. Whether through measurable physical signals or more subtle energies, vibration is a language the body understands.

A key principle in vibrational healing is **resonance**—when the frequency of one object causes another to vibrate in sync, much like a tuning fork to a musical string instrument. In healing, resonance helps the body remember its natural rhythm. Surgery, immune responses, and even deep emotional release—all reflect this principle of disruption followed by reconnection and reorganisation.

When all our bodily systems are in sync, we experience good health. But when this delicate balance is disturbed, illness can take hold. Understanding the role of vibration in health may open new doors to innovative approaches to healing and well-being.

Swedish vibrations—a gentle revolution in treatment

During a recent visit to a fascia treatment clinic in Sweden, I was introduced to a gentle but powerful form of vibrational therapy that's been quietly changing lives. Designed to treat musculo-skeletal conditions like frozen shoulder, chronic back pain, and post-whiplash symptoms, it's not flashy—but the results speak for themselves.

What sets this approach apart is its scope. Instead of zeroing in on a single painful spot, therapists use a handheld device to deliver rhythmic pulses—between 400 and 1,200 per minute—into the body's fascial system. Fascia, that endlessly weaving, body-wide connective-tissue network, responds remarkably well to this subtle input. By releasing restrictions and restoring the body's vibrational harmony, the therapy often results in reduced pain, improved mobility, and a feeling of integration many patients haven't experienced in years.

And the results? Genuinely impressive. A 2019 study by Borg

et al. looked at the effects of this therapy on people with frozen shoulder. After just three sessions over five weeks:

- 87% improved their shoulder range of motion by at least 30 degrees.
- 52% gained 60 degrees or more.
- 30% regained full movement.
- 61% reported better sleep.

These results challenge the old belief that frozen shoulder takes months—or even years—to resolve. Rather than fighting the body, this approach seems to listen to it.

But therapists don't just treat the shoulder—they treat the system. Guided by the body's myofascial meridians (those long lines of connective tissue that thread from head to toe), sessions often include gentle work on the feet, abdomen, back, and even the head. The effect is a kind of system-wide reset, influencing not just biomechanics but also nervous system regulation and overall wellbeing.

The clinic also encourages supportive lifestyle shifts: hydration, rest, movement, nutrition, and emotional balance. These aren't extras—they're part of the model itself. Everything supports the fascia. Everything matters.

The practitioners I met were not only skilled but deeply invested in their clients' progress. Many of them spoke with quiet pride about people who had arrived feeling stuck and left with renewed hope and movement. This fascia-aware, whole-body approach doesn't just mask symptoms—it goes after the vibrational and structural imbalances that create them.

Not just for humans …

Perhaps most surprising is how seamlessly this method has translated to animals. Adapted versions of the vibration device are being used to support recovery, relaxation, and mobility in horses and dogs. Several competitive equestrian teams have even credited fascial vibration therapy with improving performance—for both horse and rider. Given fascia's vital role in balance, coordination, and energy flow, it makes sense that the benefits would span species.

Looking ahead

Fascial vibration therapy isn't just a new tool—it represents a new way of thinking. Instead of asking, *"How do we fix what's broken?"*, it invites a deeper question: *"How can we help the whole body find its way back to balance?"*

As research continues to reveal fascia's role in systemic health and subtle communication, therapies like this may take their place not just on the fringes but at the heart of mainstream care. And as we learn to listen to the body's vibrational language, we may discover that healing is not only possible—it may be beautifully, rhythmically natural.

The Boundless Body

09

*"If you want to find the secrets of the universe, think
in terms of energy, frequency and vibration."*
—Nikola Tesla

What makes someone alive?

One moment, a person is thinking, feeling, moving—and the next, they are still. Their body remains, unchanged in appearance, yet something essential is missing. What is it that animates us, beyond muscles and nerves? What gives rise to awareness, movement, sensation, and emotion?

Across time and cultures, people have sensed and worked with this unseen force. Some call it *qi, prana, life force,* or *biofield energy*. Others speak of spirit, consciousness, or a single, overarching creative principle (like a universal mind)—the source of all that is, was, and will be.

Call it what you like, the core idea is the same: something beyond the physical is fundamental to being human.

The many names of life force across cultures

Throughout history, cultures around the world have recognised a vital force that animates and sustains life. While the names and interpretations vary, the core idea remains the same: life is

Names for life force across cultures

A selection of terms used in different traditions to describe the vital energy believed to animate living beings.

powered by energy—often unseen—that connects body, mind, and spirit. This sort of energy doesn't always make things *move* in a mechanical sense, but it carries information, intention, and intelligence.

NAME	ORIGIN	DESCRIPTION
Name	Origin	Description
Ātman	Hinduism	Inner self, divine essence, or soul
BARAKA	Islamic mysticism	Spiritual blessing or life force
Chi/Qi	Traditional Chinese Medicine	Vital energy flowing through meridians
Élan Vital	Philosophy	Creative life force driving evolution
Entelechy	Aristotle/philosophy	Inner force guiding growth and purpose
Holy Spirit	Christianity	Divine presence or force animating and guiding life
Huaca	Andean traditions	Sacred power in people, places, and objects
Ka	Ancient Egypt	Life essence or spiritual double
Ki	Japanese culture	Universal energy, similar to qi
Mana	Polynesian traditions	Supernatural force in people and nature
Mauri	Māori worldview	Life force linking people, land, and spirit
Megbe	Ituri Pygmies (Africa)	Animating energy connecting community and spirit
Numen	Ancient Roman religion	Divine presence or spiritual force
Odic Force	Esoteric science	Hypothetical life-linked energy
Orenda	Iroquois tradition	Invisible power within all living things
Orgone	Wilhelm Reich	Bioenergetic force in living beings
Pneuma	Ancient Greece	Breath of life, animating spirit
Prana	Hinduism/yoga	Life energy regulated through breath
Ruach	Hebrew traditions	Spirit, breath, or divine wind
Sekhem	Ancient Egypt	Spiritual might or inner power
Telesma	Hermeticism	Hidden force linking matter and spirit
Vital Force	Homeopathy/naturopathy	Self-organising life energy
Wakan	Lakota (North America)	Sacred energy that flows through everything
Yesod	Kabbalah (Jewish mysticism)	Energetic foundation linking soul to physical world

These names point to a profound insight: that being alive isn't just about physical processes. It's also about subtle patterns, connections, and meaning. And it's okay if some of this feels unfamiliar—it's not about believing everything; it's about being open to exploring new possibilities.

Health as wholeness

Many healing traditions have recognised that energy is part of what makes us whole. Modern anatomy focuses on bones, muscles, organs—what we can see, measure, and name. But what if we add energy to that picture?

Subtle energy anatomy isn't meant to replace physical anatomy. It's an extension of it—adding depth to how we understand illness, healing, and human experience.

Historically, before modern science took centre stage, health was often seen as a balance between physical, mental, emotional, and spiritual elements. From Hippocrates to Galen to traditional Chinese, Ayurvedic, and Indigenous systems, there was a deep respect for the *unseen*.

But about 400 years ago, a shift happened. Science and spirit parted ways. Philosopher René Descartes famously separated mind from body, and from then on, medicine focused on what could be dissected, seen, or quantified. Much was gained. But something was lost, too.

We're still learning to talk about energy, emotion, and consciousness in scientific terms—but that doesn't mean they aren't real.

Subtle energy—an ancient idea, a modern mystery

As author Cyndi Dale writes, "We are made of energy ... information that vibrates." From atoms to thought patterns, from skin to music—everything vibrates. What differs is the *frequency* and *amplitude*.

So why can't we always detect subtle energy with the same tools we use for sound or electricity? Possibly because it exists beyond the bandwidth of our current instruments—just as ultraviolet light, X-rays, and radio waves did before technology advanced.

Subtle energy may be imperceptible to most of our senses, but so are gravity, magnetic fields, and thoughts. Lack of measurement doesn't equal lack of existence.

The drop in the ocean—understanding energy's complexity

"The whole universe appears as a dynamic web of inseparable energy patterns ... Thus we are not separated parts of a whole. We are whole." —Barbara Ann Brennan

Imagine a scientist releasing a single drop of water into a water-filled glass container. The ripples are small, neat, and easily observed. Instruments can track the wave patterns and predict how they behave.

Now, imagine that same drop falling into the ocean during a rainstorm.

Waves crash and wind howls across the surface. Beneath, deep currents twist and swirl in unseen patterns. Tides rise and fall with the pull of the moon. The ocean is alive—shaped by salinity, temperature, marine life, seasonal shifts, and storms that haven't yet arrived.

That single drop—along with its countless rainy companions—merges with the whole. Its motion is no longer traceable or measurable. But it's still there, still part of the ocean—deeply interconnected, constantly moving, shaped by forces far greater than one ripple.

Does that mean we give up trying to understand it?

Not at all. But it means we need to *simplify* our models and expand our imagination. Just as scientists study the ocean one current at a time, we can explore subtle energy layer by layer— even if we never see the whole picture at once.

Subtle perception

"Subtle energies are higher levels of energy beginning just beyond our normal perceptive abilities … [they] are the blueprint of denser forms of matter and energy, the energy matrix out of which our perceptible universe is manifested … Around and within living creatures, including man, subtle energies are seen as an aura, reflecting the health, personality, and spirituality of the individual." —John Davidson

While most people rely on the five senses—sight, hearing, touch, taste, and smell—many traditions acknowledge that human perception extends beyond them. Some people experience brief moments of heightened awareness. Others develop these subtle senses through practice.

Personally, I've had fleeting glimpses—moments of sudden clarity or deep knowing that weren't logical but felt completely true. They left me open to the possibility that subtle perception is a natural, if poorly understood, part of being human.

Common forms of subtle sensing

A simplified overview of non-ordinary perception as described in various traditions.

TYPE	DESCRIPTION
Intuition	A gut feeling or inner knowing without conscious reasoning. Can arrive as flashes of insight.
Clairvoyance	"Clear seeing"—inner vision or imagery beyond the physical. Sometimes described as dream-like.
Clairaudience	"Clear hearing"—hearing inner sounds, words, or tones without an external source.
Clairsentience	"Clear feeling"—sensing energy, emotions, or physical sensations from people or environments.
Clairalience	"Clear smelling"—perceiving scents with no physical source, often linked to memory or spirit.
Clairgustance	"Clear tasting"—phantom tastes not related to food or drink.
Clairtangency	Also called psychometry—receiving impressions by touching objects or people.
Claircognisance	"Clear knowing"—unshakeable knowledge that arrives fully formed.
Empathy	Feeling or absorbing others' emotions, often without words or cues—closely related to clairsentience.
Presentience	A subtle sense of something about to happen; often experienced as a physical sensation, inner unease, or anticipatory knowing before an event unfolds.

As scientific interest in consciousness and energy grows, researchers are beginning to explore how subtle energies might interact with our physiology. Some propose that energy operates on a spectrum—much wider than the tiny band of frequencies we currently call "measurable".

To quote Dale again: *"It's not supernatural, paranormal, or scary—it's just energy."*

Subtle energy anatomy

For thousands of years, cultures have mapped subtle energy systems. Each model reflects a different worldview—but many share common features. These structures aren't physical in the way that nerves and bones are, but they offer useful ways to understand how energy might flow through and around the body.

Every form of healthcare rests on a model of the body. Modern medicine is grounded in *physical anatomy*. Energy-based systems rest on *subtle anatomy*.

To understand subtle anatomy, we need to step beyond the limits of linear space and location. As author Cyndi Dale explains:

> "... subtle energy structures interface between the physical body and the subtle energies (and their domains). Subtle energy structures differ in many ways from biological structures ... you cannot speak of a subtle energy structure such as a field as being located in only one place, such as out of the body. While physical bodies are restricted to one place, the subtle field penetrates every particle of the body and extends beyond it ... Subtle energies, rule breakers that they are, can stretch—and sometimes completely ignore—time and space, change form at will, and occupy many places at once."

For a deeper dive, *The Subtle Body* by Cyndi Dale (2009) is a comprehensive guide to energy systems across global traditions.

Subtle energy structures—five ways to understand the invisible body

Here's a simplified overview of five commonly described subtle energy structures:

1. Fields
These are energy environments that surround and permeate the body. The biofield is one well-known example, but many traditions describe multiple energetic layers that extend well beyond the skin—each with its own function and frequency.

2. Planes

Planes are levels of consciousness or realms of existence. Spiritual systems often refer to planes such as the physical, emotional, mental, astral, and causal—each representing a distinct vibrational frequency or mode of experience.

3. Channels

These are pathways through which life force (or energy) flows. In Traditional Chinese Medicine, they're called *meridians*; in Ayurveda, they're known as *nadis*.

The three principal nadis—*ida*, *pingala*, and *sushumna*—run along the spine and help regulate physical, mental, and emotional energy.

4. Dimensions

In science, dimensions refer to the measurable frameworks of time and space. In metaphysical contexts, they often describe expanded states of awareness or alternate levels of reality—realms that lie beyond our usual sensory perception.

5. Bodies

Subtle energy bodies are like invisible organs of energy. They receive, translate, and transmit life force throughout the human matrix—the interconnected field of subtle and physical elements that make up who we are. A familiar example is the *chakra system*—spinning energy centres aligned along the spine that influence both emotional states and physical organs. Other models, such as the *sephiroth* of Jewish Kabbalah, describe energy movement through spiritual "spheres". While the names and visuals vary, the core idea remains consistent: these energy bodies form a vital bridge between the subtle and physical.

Human matrix. A term used in this book to describe the full, interconnected field of physical, emotional, and subtle energy that makes up a human being. The human matrix includes everything from tissues and fluids to energy fields, chakras, and patterns of consciousness—it's the living blueprint that shapes how we feel, function, and heal.

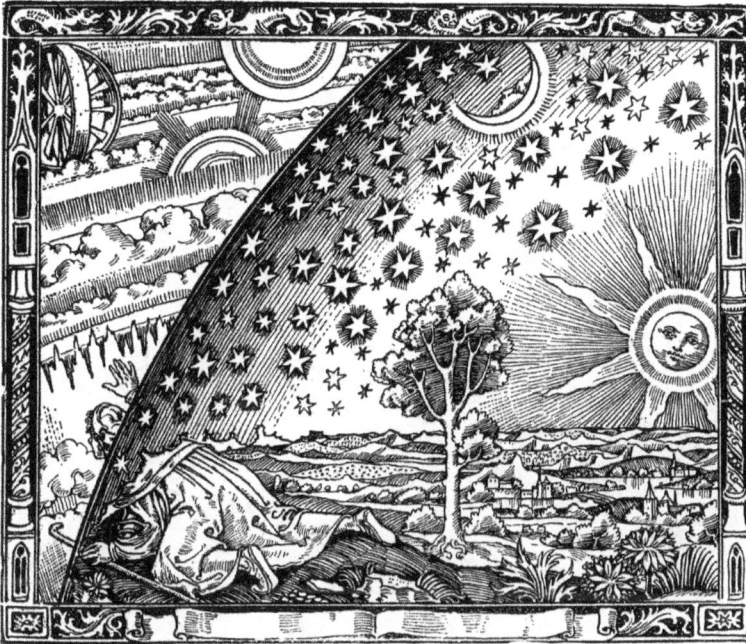

**Flammarion Engraving
(c. 1888, artist unknown)**

This famous image symbolises humanity's curiosity and drive to explore what lies beyond appearances. The figure's journey through the sky's boundary mirrors our movement through layers of consciousness, energy, and experience—much like the structures described in this chapter. It invites us to peek beyond the visible veil and consider what might lie just outside our current perception.

A helpful analogy

Think of your body like a **smartphone connected to an invisible network:**

- **Chakras** are like signals—they translate different kinds of energy (emotional, mental, spiritual, physical).
- **Nadis and meridians** are like the internal wiring and data pathways—keeping energy flowing where it's needed.
- **Other systems**—like **sephiroth or acupuncture maps**— are specialised apps that work on different layers of the network.

When your energy system is strong and flowing well, everything functions smoothly. Your messages get through. Your system stays updated. You stay *online* and in balance.

Subtle Energy Map of the Yogic Body

This intricate 19th-century Tibetan image, attributed to the prophet Ratnasara, illustrates the nadis—subtle energy channels said to carry prana (life force) throughout the body. It reflects core aspects of subtle energy anatomy as understood in classical yogic traditions. The Sanskrit title at the top reads *Prāṇāyāma*, referring to breath control practices that direct the movement of *prana* through these channels. The many letters scattered throughout the diagram aren't random: they represent syllables or *bija* (seed) sounds associated with different energy points and qualities of breath. This energetic map, later reproduced in Oschman (2003), symbolises an ancient model of inner flow, consciousness, and transformation—inviting viewers to explore the layers of experience that lie beneath physical form.

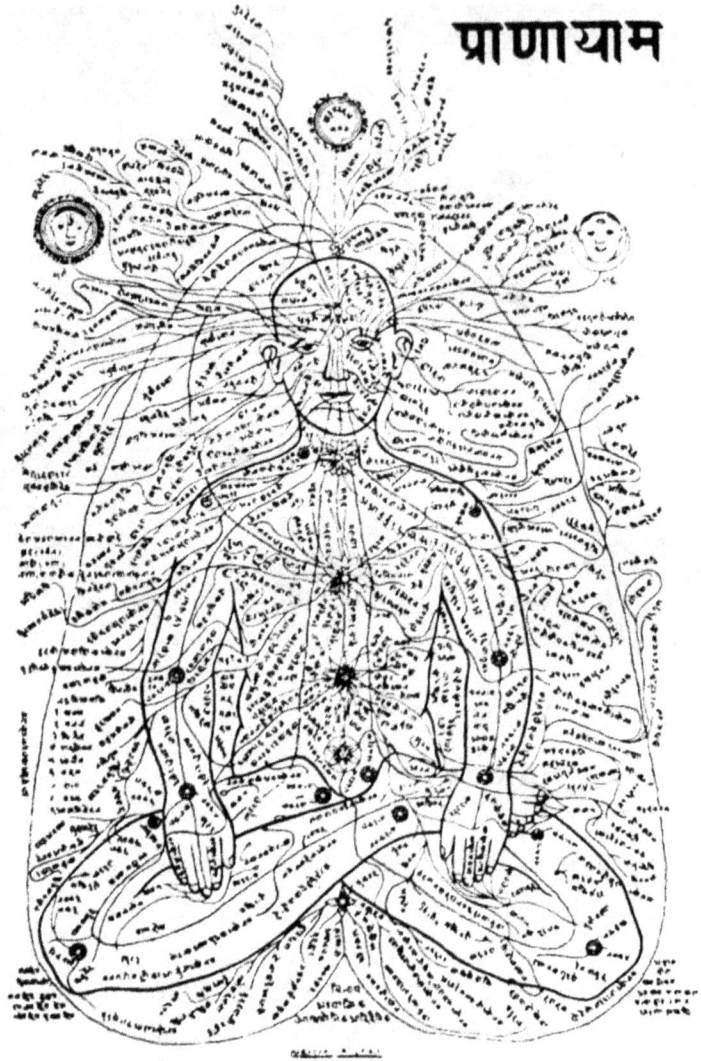

Interfaces—where energy meets structure

"The soul of man with all the streams of pure living water seems to dwell in the fascia of his body" —A. T. Still (1899)

Fascia plays a pivotal role in this flow. It surrounds and supports nerves, vessels, and meridians—acting as a generator, conduit, and reservoir of energy. Well-hydrated fascia contains structured water, with charge-separating properties that may influence electromagnetic signalling and cellular health.

Fascia isn't just passive scaffolding. It's a *living, dynamic network*—one that transports, transforms, and amplifies energy in ways we're only beginning to understand. Some have called fascia the "**skin of the spirit**"—a tangible, intelligent interface through which life energy is conducted, expressed, and perceived.

Emerging science supports the idea that fascia conducts not just mechanical and electrical signals but potentially even *subtle energetic* information. Its piezoelectric properties, its fluid matrix, and its whole-body continuity all point to fascia as a central interface between the physical and energetic.

A personal reflection

One of the most powerful descriptions of fascia I've ever encountered came from a dear friend—a Māori Miri Miri practitioner—who spoke from a lineage of deep embodied knowledge. Her words, shared before her passing, continue to resonate in my heart and my work:

"It's impossible for me to describe fascia in scientific terms because I cannot separate ideas of its physical and energetic structure, genealogy, history, and environment. So, for me and my ancestors, there's an emphasis on the flow of waters—not just blood, but water of the land. Whose waters flow through these veins? Where do you come from? Fascia takes on the life of everything, so there is no distinction between fascia and the whole. It is a hologram of essence, of the whole. Fascia and the body are not separate; they are part of the universal whole."

These words remind us that fascia is not simply a biological structure—it is part of the Earth, of story, of ancestry. Through it, we many come to remember that healing is not just restoration—it is *reconnection.*

(With heartfelt thanks to the late Miri Miri practitioner who shared this wisdom with me, and to the ancestors who allowed her to speak it.)

How Can We Improve Our Health and Wellness?

10

"One size does not fit all." —Frank Zappa

We all want to feel as healthy and well as we can. But what do the words associated with that—*health, wellness, healing*—actually mean?

Many people think of health as being free from illness. But health also implies *wholeness*—not just the absence of disease but a state of balance and vitality. Healing, in turn, is the process of *becoming whole* again. It doesn't just mean fixing something that's broken. It means reconnecting what's been separated—physically, emotionally, socially, or spiritually.

That "more elsewhere" might include everything from subtle energies and emotional integration to our connection with nature, the cosmos, community, and purpose. Healing, in this broader view, can't be reduced to physical repair alone. It happens across many layers—physical, mental, emotional, environmental, social, and spiritual—and is shaped by how we understand the body in the first place.

Has there been a time when you felt physically healed but not quite whole—or vice versa? What helped you restore your sense of balance?

"A person may be made whole, but not a whole thing. There is more elsewhere." —Sheri Tepper (1985)

Different models, different meanings

How we care for the body depends on how we see the body.

If we view the body as a machine, illness becomes a mechanical fault—and healthcare becomes a matter of finding and fixing the broken parts and processes. This view underpins most Western medicine: precise, technical, and often brilliant in acute intervention.

But if we see the body as a living, dynamic, interconnected whole—a flowing human matrix of matter, energy, memory, and meaning—then healing becomes something more expansive. It's not just about the treatment. It's about restoring connection, balance, and flow across all layers of the self.

This chapter focuses on *professional healthcare*: care delivered by trained practitioners using various models of the body. The next chapter will explore *self-care* and *self-treatment*—approaches to wellness that put more power in our own hands.

Fixing vs. healing

So how do we navigate the difference between short-term solutions and deeper transformation?

It's important to distinguish between *fixing* and *healing*.

Fixing is usually about solving a specific problem. Something's gone wrong, and we want to get things back to how they were before things turned to custard (as we say in this part of the world). It's practical, targeted, and often symptom-focused.

Healing is broader and deeper. It may involve fixing, but it also includes growth, adaptation, and transformation. Healing doesn't always mean returning to the *same*—it can mean becoming *more whole* than before. And ultimately, healing is something *you* do; no one else can do it for you.

As author and healer Steve Nobel puts it:

"A healer does not actually heal. A healer facilitates healing vibrations that the client can choose to accept or not. Thus the 'success' of any healing is in the hands of the receiver."

Health vs. wellbeing—what's the difference?

Think of **health** as the mechanics—your body's systems working the way they should. Health can be measured: blood pressure, iron levels, joint mobility, pain scores. It's functional and important.

But wellbeing is your lived experience of being alive. It includes your emotions, sense of purpose, energy levels, relationships, creativity—even your connection to something greater. You can be healthy on paper but still feel unwell. And sometimes people with serious illness can feel deeply well in spirit—as I often saw when I worked in a hospice.

A simple metaphor:

- **Health** is a well-maintained car.
- **Wellbeing** is enjoying the ride.

To truly thrive, we need both!

Professional health care—a wide spectrum

Professional healthcare spans a wide spectrum—because healing isn't one-size-fits-all. It includes all forms of health support provided by trained and qualified practitioners—from mainstream medicine (like doctors, nurses, and surgeons) to allied and complementary professions such as physiotherapy, massage therapy, osteopathy, acupuncture, and naturopathy.

Most professional healthcare systems are built on *evidence-based practice*. This means treatments are guided by research, clinical expertise, and patient outcomes. In theory, this ensures care is safe, effective, and consistent—though in reality, this ideal isn't always achieved.

But this raises a deeper question: *"What kind of evidence counts?"*

Randomised controlled trials—often conducted in highly controlled settings—are considered the gold standard of scientific evidence. But there is also great value in thousands of years of lived observation: healing practices refined through cultural transmission, trial and error, and close attention to what works in real-life, everyday situations.

Both approaches bring something important to the table. Who's to say one form of evidence should always outrank the other? Or that we shouldn't combine them—and benefit from both at the same time?

Moreover, "evidence-based" doesn't always mean relevant to *you*. Many studies focus on populations that may not reflect your age, gender, culture, or way of life. Much of medical research has historically centred on young, biologically male Western bodies—leaving women, gender-diverse people, and non-Western perspectives underrepresented.

That's why context matters. So does lived experience. Real-world care needs more than just data—it needs relevance, respect, and room for multiple truths. When we draw from both science and story, healthcare becomes more inclusive, more responsive—more human and humane.

True healthcare honours data and story, science and soul.It listens to research—but also to the person in front of it.

One size doesn't fit all.

Healing, like humans, is rarely one-size-fits-anything.

That's why many people seek care from multiple sources. They might consult a GP for diagnosis, work with a physiotherapist for movement support, and turn to a naturopath, rongoā Māori healer, or acupuncturist for a more holistic or energy-aware approach. Some are drawn to the confidence and clarity of mainstream medicine. Others choose systems of care that reflect their cultural heritage, personal values, or lived experience.

The limits of standardisation

Standardisation has its place—it promotes safety and consistency. But it can introduce rigidity. Health systems built on fixed protocols may overlook individuals whose needs don't match the average.

This isn't a criticism of practitioners—most are doing their best within the frameworks they've learned and work under. But these frameworks sometimes emphasise symptom control over root-cause exploration, and fragmentation over whole-person care.

Acute medical care is often life-saving. But when it comes to chronic conditions, subtle imbalance, emotional distress, or energetic depletion, a more integrative approach can offer something extra.

Different models, different strengths

To illustrate how varied healthcare approaches can be, here are just a few contrasting examples:

HEALTH FOCUS	MAINSTREAM EXAMPLE	COMPLEMENTARY/ ALTERNATIVE EXAMPLE
Cellular health	IV (intravenous) nutrition therapy	Homeopathic cell salts
Tissue repair	Stem cell injections	Prolotherapy
Organ support	Dialysis for kidney function	Herbal medicine for liver detoxification
Musculoskeletal health	Orthopaedic surgery	Chiropractic adjustments
Fascia/connective tissue	Steroid therapy, physiotherapy	Myofascial release therapy, Rolfing/ structural integration
Mental and emotional health	Psychotherapy/psychiatry	Energy psychology - e.g., EFT (emotionally focused therapy), EMDR (eye movement desensitising and reprocessing therapy)
Energy healing	PEMF (pulsed electromagnetic field energy), TMS (transcranial magnetic stimulation)	Reiki, qigong, acupuncture

Professional healthcare—strengths and shortcomings

Like any system, professional healthcare has both strengths and limitations. Acknowledging both can help us make wise, compassionate choices about the care we seek—and the care we offer others.

> **PROS:**
> ✅ Expert care from highly trained professionals.
> ✅ Advanced diagnostics and treatments.
> ✅ Emergency and acute care capabilities.
> ✅ Regulated ethical standards.
> ✅ Strong support for complex or life-threatening conditions.

CONS:

- ✗ Symptom-focused rather than root-cause oriented.
- ✗ Expensive or inaccessible for some.
- ✗ Fragmented care across body systems.
- ✗ May overly rely on medication and procedures.
- ✗ Less emphasis on lifestyle, prevention, and empowerment.

In a complex world, healing often means weaving together many threads. What matters most is that the approach feels right for the whole person—not just their symptoms.

Acupuncture—bridging traditions

A growing number of healthcare systems now include acupuncture as part of integrative care. Its effects have been widely studied, with research confirming its ability to reduce pain, regulate the nervous system, and enhance overall quality of life.

While acupuncture originated in Traditional Chinese Medicine, it has increasingly found its place within evidence-informed frameworks. It is now recognised and practised by physiotherapists, GPs, and specialists in many Western countries. In this way, acupuncture becomes a bridge between different ways of seeing the body—honouring both energetic wisdom and physiological science.

It reminds us that healing need not be exclusive to one tradition. It can draw on the best of many.

Lisa's story: integrating professions, expanding healing

Lisa began her professional journey as a sports physiotherapist, firmly grounded in Western biomedical training. For 14 years, she worked with athletes, muscles, joints, and injuries—focused on physical function, evidence-based techniques, and results. It was a world of clear goals, treatment protocols, and measurable outcomes.

But over time, something began to shift. The more she worked with patients, the more she sensed that the standard tools didn't always address the *whole* story. Pain wasn't always just about the injured part—it was tangled with lifestyle, stress, unresolved emotion, and deeper imbalances that didn't fit into the clinical checklists.

Out of curiosity, Lisa attended a short acupuncture course tailored for physiotherapists. It was her first real encounter with a completely different way of thinking about the body—not as a collection of parts but as a living, flowing, interconnected system. She began weaving some of what she learned into her sessions, and her patients responded.

And then came the turning point.

While out trail running in a nearby forest, Lisa was accidentally sprayed by an aerial top-dressing plane releasing a biological insecticide—part of a government programme to control the spread of the painted apple moth. Although officially deemed safe for humans, some studies suggested it could cause adverse reactions in sensitive individuals. Lisa was one of them.

Within days, she developed severe eczema. The constant itching, inflammation, discomfort, and visibly damaged skin were both physically and emotionally draining. Her dermatologist prescribed prednisone and steroid creams—but Lisa, ever the health-conscious professional, was reluctant to rely on medication long-term. She wanted a solution that addressed the root cause—not just the symptoms.

On a friend's recommendation, she turned to Traditional Chinese Medicine (TCM).

She began regular acupuncture sessions, combined with dietary changes and lifestyle adjustments. Over time, her symptoms eased. But it wasn't until she was introduced to Chinese herbal medicine that a deeper shift occurred. Within three months, the eczema was gone.

The transformation reshaped how Lisa understood healing—and reignited her curiosity.

Inspired by her own recovery, Lisa enrolled in a four-year acupuncture programme at a respected TCM college. Many of her classmates came from Western health professions—like massage, midwifery, and nursing—and were embarking on acupuncture as a second career. After graduating, she worked in an integrative health clinic before opening her own acupuncture practice, which she's now run successfully for more than 15 years.

Although she maintains her physiotherapy registration, Lisa explains, "I always use acupuncture—with every patient." At first, her caseload was varied: clients with cancer-related symptoms, fertility challenges, digestive issues, and emotional distress. But due to her physiotherapy background, she quickly became known for her work with musculoskeletal conditions—back pain, neck pain, joint injuries.

"It's not what I originally had in mind," she says with a smile, "but I'm happy with it. People come in for pain relief, and then sometimes we address things like sleep, digestion, or blood pressure. It naturally expands."

Lisa now blends evidence-based physiotherapy knowledge with TCM's energetic principles. Her sessions typically begin with acupuncture (which helps patients relax and often provides immediate relief), followed by gentle hands-on work: massage, acupressure, mobilisations, or stretching.

When new clients ask how acupuncture works, Lisa adapts her explanation to suit their worldview: "The traditional Chinese believe there's an energy called qi. If it's blocked, we help restore the flow so the body can heal."

"But if someone's more science-minded, I'll say: inserting needles triggers the body's healing response—blood flow, serotonin, hormones, immune factors. I could explain the science, but most people just want to know it works."

Lisa didn't grow up with alternative medicine. Her parents, both European immigrants, firmly believed in conventional healthcare. Acupuncture had never been on her radar—until conventional care couldn't help her. What initially felt like a crisis turned out to be a catalyst. In her words: "At the time, the eczema felt like the worst thing that had ever happened to me. I had to quit a well-paying job. I had a big mortgage. I was miserable. But now? I see it as the best thing that ever happened. It completely changed the trajectory of my life."

A practitioner of two worlds

Lisa is now professionally registered with both the New Zealand Board of Physiotherapy and the Chinese Medical Council, and she remains a member of both professional associations. Staying current with both helps her honour the full range of her training and offer clients care that's grounded, integrated, and authentic.

Her story is a reminder that professional healthcare doesn't have to be either/or. It can be both/and. Science and spirit. Western logic and Eastern flow. Knowledge and curiosity. Experience and openness to the unknown.

Lisa's journey shows us that healing doesn't have to be confined to one system, one belief, or one pathway. The most powerful care often arises when we allow different forms of knowledge—scientific, cultural, energetic, embodied—to meet.

In a world of complexity, integration may be our greatest form of medicine.

How Can I Improve My Own Health and Wellness?

11

"Take care of your body. It's the only place you have to live in. If you don't make time for wellness, you'll be forced to make time for your illness"
—Robin Sharma

Many people today are asking this very question—*"How can I improve my health and wellness?"* And for good reason. With rising healthcare costs, long wait times, and growing interest in preventative approaches, more of us are wondering what we can do to stay well—or get better—on our own terms. This chapter explores that space: the power of self-care and self-treatment.

A personal note

I grew up in the countryside, the eldest of three children born to schoolteacher parents. Healthcare wasn't a regular concern in our home—not until we moved to the city after my father's tragic death. He'd developed a severe strep throat infection while leading a remote school camp. With no easy access to medical care and his strong sense of duty to his students, he stayed in the field instead of seeking help. Antibiotics could have saved him.

Until then, we'd managed our health at home, just like many of our rural neighbours. Going to the doctor wasn't part of daily life. We ate fresh, homegrown produce, drank milk from local farms, and made most of our food from scratch. We played outdoors, often barefoot, and got plenty of sleep. Television didn't arrive until I was ten, and mobile phones hadn't been imagined.

At the first sign of illness, we were tucked into bed with instructions to rest and drink fluids. Measles, chicken pox, and mumps were all handled at home with calm reassurance. Remedies were simple: lemon and honey drinks, homemade broths, and a tin of antiseptic "pink ointment." Doctor visits were rare—and only when absolutely necessary.

Later, raising my own children in the city, I carried many of these practices forward. But when they started preschool and brought home a cycle of illness, I realised health wasn't just about individual choices—it was also about context. Not everyone could afford to stay home to care for sick kids. Illness spread quickly. Going to the doctor had become normal and, for many, frequent.

That experience sparked a deeper curiosity. Why did people seem to rely so much on doctors and medication to stay healthy? For my own family, I began exploring some other options: naturopathy, herbal medicine, homeopathy, Reiki, massage, and organic gardening. This approach kept us mostly well. And when we needed medical care, we sought it gratefully. But the habit of staying open and curious has reshaped my life and work.

Blending traditions—healing across the spectrum

Over the years, I've explored a wide range of methods—some mainstream, some unconventional, and some that might seem a little "out there." What I've learned is simple: different approaches exist for a reason. They work.

- Just like antibiotics work.
- Just like surgery works.
- Just like physiotherapy works.
- Just like acupuncture works.
- Just like Miri Miri (traditional Māori massage) works
- Just like Reiki (energy healing) works.

Not for everyone, not every time—but often enough to matter.

Healthcare exists on a continuum. At one end, there is the expertise of trained professionals. At the other, we have our own innate capacity to care for, treat, and heal ourselves. In between are community-based healers, complementary therapists, supportive family members, and the countless ways people care for one another other in daily life.

Healing isn't about choosing one approach over another. It's about recognising what kind of care is most appropriate for *us* in each moment—and weaving them together where possible.

Self-care and self-treatment

Self-care and self-treatment are two sides of the same coin. They share a common goal: to help us feel better and stay well.

- **Self-care** refers to everyday habits that support well-being—like nourishing food, regular movement, rest, and meaningful connection.
- **Self-treatment** refers to strategies we use when something isn't quite right—like applying a home remedy, resting a sore joint, or trying a technique to ease symptoms.

Both are essential. Both are increasingly necessary in a world where access to healthcare isn't always easy or affordable. And both remind us that health is not just something we "receive" from others—it's something we grow and sustain ourselves.

Why self-care matters

People turn to self-care for many reasons:

- Healthcare access may be limited or costly.
- Natural approaches align better with their beliefs.
- Professional care doesn't always bring resolution.
- They want to feel more in control of their health.

And while the wellness industry often focuses on things to *buy*, meaningful self-care is about what you *do*. It's the daily choices that build resilience, vitality, and agency—often in quiet, unglamorous ways.

Navigating the wellness industry

Self-care is having a moment—and that's not always a good thing. Self-care isn't just about bubble baths and green smoothies. It's about taking charge of your health in small, sustainable, and meaningful ways.

Wellness is now big business: seminars, workshops, retreats, apps, supplements, skincare lines, podcasts, YouTube channels. Some are created by experts. Others by influencers with no training. Some products and services are genuinely helpful. Others are eye-wateringly expensive, unnecessary, or even misleading.

It's easy to get overwhelmed or disillusioned. That's why I favour do-it-yourself approaches—practices that are accessible, grounded, and empowering. Things you can try at home without spending a fortune. Not because they're trendy but because they've stood the test of time. There's no single "right" approach—only what works for you.

A personal turning point

That said, even the most committed self-carer sometimes needs support. A few years ago, after a winter fall on black ice led to multiple surgeries, I found myself struggling. I was older, stiffer, sitting too much, in pain. When I couldn't lift my carry-on into the overhead locker on a flight, I knew something had to change.

Enter Mandy—a fitness coach whose own recovery from a life-threatening accident had transformed her career. Formerly a radiation therapist, she'd rebuilt herself from scratch and was now helping others do the same. Her blend of evidence-informed knowledge and lived experience was exactly what I needed. Her approach didn't just address my pain—it reawakened my sense of agency.

We worked together privately over a series of 30-minute sessions. Her practical, fascia-aware advice built on what I already knew—but filled in the gaps. Six weeks later, I was lifting that carry-on. Three months in, I felt stronger, straighter, and more alive in my body.

Her "five solutions for a thriving body":

- **Move and groove**—strength and resilience.
- **Fuel**—nutrient-dense, anti-inflammatory food.
- **Hydration**—2–3 litres daily.
- **Sleep**—quality and consistency.
- **Gut microbiome**—maintain healthy balance.

Simple. Sustainable. Effective.

Benefits and pitfalls

PROS OF SELF-CARE

✅ **Empowerment**—It helps you take control of your health and well-being, giving you a sense of independence.

✅ **Prevention**—Regular self-care can help prevent many health issues from developing or worsening.

✅ **Improved mental health**—Taking time for yourself reduces stress, improves mood, and boosts emotional well-being.

✅ **Cost-effective**—Many self-care practices, like meditation or walking, are free or low-cost.

✅ **Personalised**—You can tailor your routine to suit your specific needs and preferences.

CONS OF SELF-CARE

❌ **Lack of professional guidance**—Without expert input, some practices may be ineffective or even cause harm if done incorrectly.

❌ **Overwhelm**—It can feel like there's a lot to manage, especially when juggling multiple responsibilities.

❌ **Limited results**—While valuable, self-care isn't a substitute for medical treatment in serious cases.

❌ **Inconsistency**—It's easy to fall out of rhythm with a self-care routine, especially with a busy lifestyle.

❌ **Too much focus on the individual**—Self-care matters, but so do support systems.

Self-treatment—helping yourself heal

While self-care keeps us well, self-treatment helps us get better. It involves using safe, natural, and thoughtful strategies to ease symptoms, support healing, and reduce discomfort.

Self-treatment includes lifestyle adjustments, natural

methods, and home remedies. It's about playing an active role in managing minor ailments or aiding recovery. Used wisely, it complements—but does not replace—professional care.

When used with caution and common sense, self-treatment can:

- Prevent expensive visits or long waits.
- Promote quicker recovery.
- Alleviate discomfort.
- Foster deeper body awareness.

But if symptoms persist, worsen, or feel unusual, it's always best to consult a professional healthcare provider. Use common sense. If something feels off, don't ignore it.

Self-treatment is especially useful for:

- Soft tissue pain.
- Swelling or inflammation.
- Minor injuries (like bruises, stings, and sprains).
- Stress and nervous system regulation.
- Boosting energy and mood.

You don't need fancy tools. Your hands, a hot water bottle, some elastic tape, your breath—and a little patience—can go a long way.

Some simple self-treatment options include:

- Balancing rest and movement.
- Using hot water bottles, cold compresses, or contrast baths.
- Soothing sore areas with your hands.
- Percussion (gently using a soft fist or massage gun).
- Applying elastic tape to ease tension and improve fluid flow.

Remember, self-treatment isn't about pushing through pain. It's about listening, supporting, and helping the body shift.

Because self-treatment isn't widely discussed—often due to concerns about safety and liability—it can seem unfamiliar. But many of our grandparents, neighbours, and community elders used it as a first line of care. Ask them what helped. Their answers might surprise you.

And remember, some healthcare professionals can offer excellent advice here too—especially those with a holistic or integrative mindset. A physio might teach you safe stretching. A massage therapist might show postural tips. A naturopath might recommend herbs. Their insights can complement your own observations beautifully.

Pros and cons of self-treatment

PROS:

✅ **Empowerment**—Encourages confidence and a deeper relationship you're your body.

✅ **Cost-effective**—Many options are low-cost and may reduce the need for medical visits.

✅ **Convenience**—You can treat minor issues quickly at home.

✅ **Prevention**—Regular self-treatment can reduce the chance of small issues becoming big ones.

✅ **Body awareness**—Builds intuition and knowledge about your own system.

CONS:

❌ **Overconfidence**—It's easy to overestimate what can be managed alone.

❌ **Misdiagnosis**—Without training, symptoms might be misunderstood.

❌ **Delayed care**—Relying on self-treatment too long may delay proper help.

- ✖ **Inconsistent results**—What works well for one person might not for another.
- ✖ **Misuse**—Overusing remedies or tools (like essential oils or stretching) can backfire.

Safety first

Both self-care and self-treatment can be powerful tools for supporting your health. But always exercise caution. If something doesn't feel right, if you're unsure, or if symptoms linger—reach out for help. Your health is too important to gamble with.

Neither of these approaches is a replacement for professional care. The best self-care is informed, grounded, and humble enough to know when to ask for support.

The big picture

Healing is deeply personal. There's no one-size-fits-all solution. Some people feel better with acupuncture. Others with medication. Some need yoga. Others thrive with resistance training or intermittent fasting.

The most important thing? Stay curious. Try things. Keep what helps. Let go of what doesn't. Give yourself permission to adapt as you grow.

When we invest in our health—not just to fix it, but to care for it—we become stronger, more resilient, and more connected to our lives.

That's what self-care is really about.

Coming up next: We'll explore the bigger picture—what all of this means for our communities, health systems, and the future of care. Because when individuals begin to take charge of their own healing, the ripple effects can be profound.

Where to From Here?

12

"Health problems are part of life.
Healthcare problems shouldn't be."
—Roadside billboard

Across the world, healthcare systems are under strain. Patients wait too long to be seen. Practitioners burn out. Costs spiral. Solutions are trialled, debated, funded—and often fall short. We've tried fixing the system from within: more money, more buildings, more staff, new policies. Yet something deeper still seems off.

As Einstein once said, *"We cannot solve our problems with the same thinking we used when we created them."* If we want different results, we need different thinking—not just about healthcare but also about the body at the heart of it.

That shift in thinking begins with how we perceive, understand, and relate to the body itself.

Rethinking the body

For centuries, Western medicine has relied on the image of the body as a machine—a complicated assemblage of separate parts with separate problems and separate fixes. This model gave us incredible tools: surgery, antibiotics, vaccines, and specialist care. But it also left gaps. It fragmented and distorted our understanding of health. It prioritised parts over people, symptoms over stories, and correction over connection.

We've forgotten that there are *many* ways to understand a body—and that all of them have served different cultural and historical moments. As explored in Chapter 2, a body can be:

- A tangible, physical form
- A lifeless cadaver used for teaching
- A collection of organs, tissues, and cells
- A selection of "important" parts—excluding those deemed less significant (like fascia)
- A biologically whole, functioning unit
- A mortal form, distinct from soul or spirit
- A human being, alive with sensation and energy
- A sacred dwelling place of consciousness

Each of these perspectives reveals something. None are wrong—but none tell the whole story. Trouble begins when we rely on just one lens—especially in the systems we build around care.

Take anatomy. It matters more than most people realise. The way we define and describe the body shapes how we treat it. Traditional anatomical models present the body as dissected and lifeless—broken down into parts. But living bodies—the ones we actually inhabit—are naturally whole, responsive, and deeply entangled with the contexts they live in. They are expressive, adaptive, and ever-changing.

Fascia, the body-wide system explored throughout this book, reminds us that we're not collections of separate parts. We're multifaceted, interconnected beings. What affects one part inevitably influences the whole.

So what might happen if we expanded our understanding—our *perception*—of the body? What if we moved beyond the machine metaphor and embraced a fascia-aware view that recognises the body as whole, alive, sensing, and inseparable from its environment?

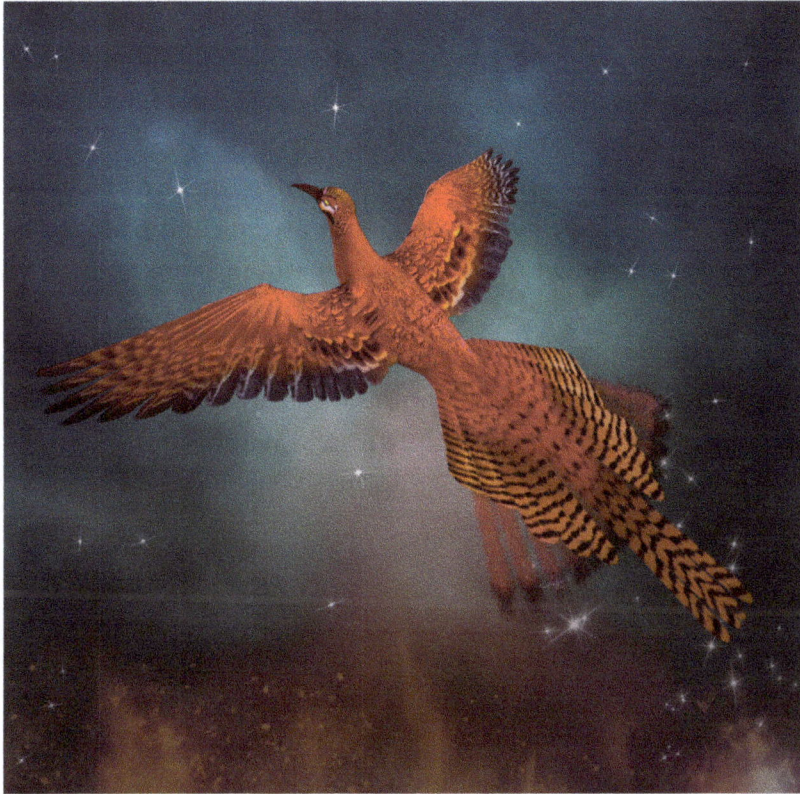

Rethinking the health system

As things stand, our healthcare systems resemble wildfire response: constantly reacting to flare-ups, pouring resources into whatever area is burning most urgently, and still unable to put the flames out entirely. The focus is emergency response—and understandably so. But in this relentless firefighting mode, we rarely pause to ask:

What caused the fire? What is fuelling it? And how can we prevent it from reigniting?

Meanwhile, the system's appetite—for money, people, technology—is insatiable. However much we feed it, it's never quite enough to meet rising demand. Everyone is doing their best, but that best isn't—and maybe never will be—enough. Because the system itself is no longer fit for purpose. We're building bigger, more expensive firebreaks, but the underlying conditions remain dry, depleted, and flammable.

Perhaps we've been patching up a system that isn't meant to be patched. Perhaps it's passed its use-by date and needs to be replaced with something fresher—something more attuned to today's world.

Like the mythical phoenix—a bird that lives for centuries, burns itself, and rises anew from the ashes—maybe our health system isn't broken so much as ready to be reborn.

A new beginning

Change of this magnitude rarely begins at the top. It's too big, too daunting. Instead, it starts from the grassroots—with the people who live within and alongside the system. It begins with a shift in perspective about what we truly need—and what we're willing to invest in.

This shift starts with reimagining healthcare not just as something done *to* us by expert others but something we engage in for ourselves, every day. For that to happen, we need to demystify anatomy. The body doesn't have to be an impossibly complex puzzle only experts can interpret. It can be understood—clearly and simply—as a living, intelligent system that its owner can get to know intimately over time.

When we see the body this way, our questions change.

From, *"What treatment will fix me?"*

To: *"How can I support my body's natural ability to heal and feel well?"*

This shift doesn't replace professional healthcare—it complements it. It lays the foundation for a more balanced model that includes:

- **Professional care** that is competent, compassionate, and collaborative
- **Community care** that is accessible, contextual, and culturally safe
- **Self-care** that is informed, supported, and trusted
- **Self-treatment** that is empowered, practical, and safe

It also broadens the cast of characters involved in healthcare—not just doctors and specialists but *also* teachers, parents, body-workers, friends, elders, and everyday individuals equipped with the tools to care for themselves and others.

The truth is, most of us aren't powerless. We can choose to live ourselves sick—or live ourselves well. Not everyone has this choice, but many of us do. And the more of us who take it, the less weight the system must carry.

What could this look like?

Imagine if:

- Every child learned about fascia, posture, breath, hydration, nutrition, and the balance between rest and movement.
- Every clinic offered guidance on safe self-treatment along-side professional care.
- Every community had access to fascia-aware education, bodywork and movement therapy.
- Every practitioner saw themselves not just as a fixer, but as a facilitator of healing and learning.

This isn't fantasy. Seeds of this vision already exist—in integra-tive clinics, community initiatives, body-literate workplaces, and empowered homes. But to grow, they need nourishing. They need people. And they need stories like yours to help them take root.

IF WE WERE TO BEGIN TO HEAL OUR HEALTH SYSTEM TODAY …

Change doesn't have to start with a grand overhaul. It can begin with small, grounded, human-centred actions. Here are three ideas:

1. A national fascia-aware self-care education campaign

Objective: Empower people to understand their bodies, manage soft tissue pain, and prevent chronic issues—before they need clinical care.

Examples:

- Co-branded campaigns with public health organisations.
- Interactive content (videos, comics, apps).
- Programmes in schools and community centres.
- Train-the-trainer sessions for educators and community leaders.

Why it matters: Builds body literacy early, encourages proactive self-care, and helps reduce strain on overwhelmed practitioners.

2. Fascia-informed practitioner upskilling initiative

Objective: Equip healthcare providers with fascia-aware knowledge and self-care strategies they can pass on to patients.

Examples:

- Subsidised continuing professional development (CPD) modules.
- Fascia content in health science and medical education.
- Liaison roles in clinics and hospitals.

Why it matters: Encourages integrative, sustainable care that bridges practitioner and patient knowledge.

3. Community-based integrative health hubs

Objective: Create local centres where people can access fascia-aware education and support from qualified guides.

Examples:

- Hubs located in clinics, libraries, or marae.
- Drop-in sessions with trained facilitators.
- Story and outcome-based research integrated into practice.

Why it matters: Models a human, scalable approach to health built on connection and trust.

These aren't top-down blueprints. They're bottom-up possibilities. And they're already partly happening—just waiting to be nurtured, expanded, and made visible.

Healing, not just fixing

"Setbacks set the stage for reinvention." —Amy Shoenthal

Pain—whether in our bodies or our health systems—is a signal. It tells us that something needs to change. Ignoring it won't help. Numbing it may buy time but doesn't address the root cause. Listening to it—that's where transformation begins.

Healing doesn't unfold in straight lines. It flows in waves. It rises from breakdown—as it did for Lisa, Mandy, Nick, and me. And it asks for courage, patience, and new ways of seeing.

We're not just waiting for a better system. We're part of what it's becoming—through the choices we make, the bodies we honour, the conversations we start, and the care we offer, to ourselves and each other.

So wherever you are in this story—practitioner, policymaker, parent, or patient—thank you for being here.

May this book be a small part of a much bigger healing. And may you remember, always:

Your body is whole. It is alive. It is shaped by, and shaping, everything around you.

It is part of a *human matrix*—an intelligent, living, sensing field where structure, sensation, and consciousness meet.

When we honour this, how we care for our bodies—and each other—can begin to shift.

And you are far more capable than you've been led to believe.

The future of healthcare doesn't just belong to institutions.

It belongs to us.

One breath, one body, one decision at a time.

Postscript

If this book has sparked something for you—thank you for journeying with me.

Your reflections, shares, and reviews truly help others find their way to this work. If you feel moved to leave a review, I'd be so grateful.

And if you're interested in bringing these ideas into your community, workplace, or event—whether through a talk, workshop, or collaborative conversation—I'd love to hear from you. You'll find contact details and further resources at sueadstrum.com.

Together, we can keep reimagining what it means to be well.

Glossary

Acupuncture — Traditional Chinese practice involving thin needles inserted into specific points on the body to balance energy flow and support healing.

Adaptability — Capacity to adjust and cope with change—vital for health and wellbeing.

Alternative therapies — Non-mainstream treatments used in place of conventional medicine.

Amplitude — Strength or intensity of a vibration or wave—how big or powerful it is.

Anatomy — Scientific study of the structure of organisms and their parts, often based on dissection and visual observation.

  – Anatomist — Person who studies and describes the structure of the human body.

  – Integrative anatomy — Combines insights from multiple disciplines—scientific, clinical, cultural, and experiential—to understand the body as a whole, living system.

  – Macroscopic (or gross) anatomy — Study of body structures visible to the naked eye, such as muscles, bones, and organs.

  – Microscopic anatomy — Study of the body's tiny structures, like cells and tissues, that require a microscope to be seen.

  – Subtle anatomy — Way of understanding the body's energy structure that includes energy fields, channels, and centres—not just physical structures.

Aponeurosis — Broad, flat sheet (tendon)of fascial (connective) tissue that attaches muscles to other muscles or bones.

Areolar tissue — Type of loose fascial (connective) tissue that fills spaces between organs, helps hold them in place, and allows them to glide easily alongside each other.

Arteries	Blood vessels that conduct blood away from the heart.
BCE (Before the Common Era)	Years before the start of the Common Era (CE), which is the same as BC (Before Christ).
Bicipital instability	Condition where the tendon of the biceps muscle (a muscle in your upper arm) is unstable.
Biofield	Energy field that surrounds and flows through the body, made up of subtle and electromagnetic signals.
Biological	Relating to living organisms or life processes. This term can be used to describe things that are part of the natural world, such as cells, plants, animals, or even ecosystems.
Biomechanics	Study of how the body moves.
Biophotons	Tiny packets of light emitted by cells, thought to help with communication.
Biotensegrity (biological tensegrity) model	Way of thinking that uses the theory of tensegrity to describe how the body, unified by fascia, moves as a whole.
Body literacy	Ability to understand, interpret, and respond to the signals of one's own body.
Body-mind	Concept that emphasizes how the body's physical condition shapes mental states, emotions, and cognition.
Body system	A group of organs, tissues, and structures that work together to carry out a major function in the body—like movement, circulation, or digestion (e.g., the musculoskeletal system, nervous system, and fascial system).
Bodywork	Range of whole-body centred treatment methods used to improve health and wellbeing.
Breathwork	Controlled breathing exercises used to calm the mind, reduce stress, and improve wellbeing.
Burnout	Physical and emotional exhaustion caused by chronic workplace stress.
Cadaver	Lifeless body, or corpse, used for medical education and research.
CE (Common Era)	Time period used in place of AD (Anno Domini).

Cell	The smallest biological structural unit.
Chakra	Spinning energy centres along the body (usually along the spine) that process and direct different kinds of energy.
Chronic disease	Long-term health conditions such as diabetes, heart disease, and autoimmune disorders that require ongoing management.
Coherence	Sense of harmony or integration within oneself and with the world around them.
Collagen (Type I)	Strong fibrous protein that is abundantly found in fascia, including tendons and ligaments.
Complementary care	Health practices used alongside conventional treatments, such as acupuncture, naturopathy, or massage.
Connective tissue	Group of tissues that connect, support, bind, or separate other parts of the body. There are two main types: **connective tissue proper** (like loose/areolar and dense connective tissue) and **specialised connective tissue** (such as fat, cartilage, bone, and even blood).
Consciousness	Awareness of thoughts, feelings, and surroundings.
Context	Situation or background in which something occurs. Influences how we perceive things.
Contrast bath	Technique involving alternating hot and cold water to stimulate circulation and reduce inflammation.
CranioSacral therapy	Gentle fascia-relating system of bodywork therapy that uses light touch to help release deep tensions in the body, eliminate pain, restore movement, and improve health and wellbeing.
Culture	Integrated and integrating social environment characterised by shared philosophies, practices, and attitudes.
Dissection	Process of (metaphorically and literally) dividing a body into parts.
Elastic tape	Flexible tape applied to the body to support joints, ease discomfort, and improve circulation or lymph flow.
Electrical energy	Energy created by the movement of charged particles, such as nerve signals.
Electromagnetic energy	Energy created when electricity and magnetism interact.

Embalming	Preserving a dead body with chemicals to protect it from decay.
Empathy	Ability to understand and share feelings with another person.
Empirical	Based on observation and evidence rather than theory.
Energy field	Non-physical space where energy is present. Some fields can be measured (like magnetic fields); others are more subtle.
Energy medicine	Healing approaches that focus on using energy fields to influence health and well-being.
Evidence-based practice	Healthcare decisions informed by clinical expertise, patient needs, and the best available research.
Fascia	Continuous, connective tissue web that surrounds and supports every part of the body, contributing to structural integrity and communication.
– A fascia (pl., fasciae)	Macroscopic piece of fascial tissue.
– Fascial tissue	Soft connective tissue.
– Fascial substance	Fascial tissue's moist, gel-like ground substance.
– Fascial system	Body-pervading web of fascial tissue with a variety of functional formats.
– Fascia-relating bodywork	Bodywork that overtly relates to the treatment of fascia.
Firefighting model	Metaphor for health systems constantly reacting to crises rather than addressing underlying causes or investing in prevention.
Frequency	How fast something vibrates—measured in cycles per second (Hertz). Higher frequencies = faster vibrations.
Frozen shoulder	Condition causing pain and stiffness in the shoulder joint.
Ground substance	Amorphous gel-like substance that surrounds and supports connective tissue cells and fibres.
Hauora	Māori term for health and wellbeing that includes physical, mental, social, and spiritual aspects of health.
Healing	Process of becoming whole again, which may include physical, emotional, mental, and spiritual restoration—not just the elimination of symptoms.

Healing vs fixing	Healing restores whole-body balance; fixing targets isolated symptoms.
Health	How well the body functions as a whole. Not just the absence of illness.
Health practitioner	Person practicing a particular healing discipline (e.g., massage).
Health professional	Paid occupational vocation that requires prolonged training and a formal qualification.
Holistic	Considering the whole of something, rather than just its parts.
Holistic health	Model of health that considers physical, mental, emotional, social, and sometimes spiritual dimensions of wellbeing—not just symptoms or conditions.
Human matrix	The interconnected field of physical and subtle elements that make up a human being. It includes tissues, fluids, energy fields, and patterns of consciousness—shaping how we feel, function, and heal.
Hydrated fascia	Well-hydrated fascia contains organised (structured) water molecules that may support energy conduction in the body.
Hydration	Keeping the body well-supplied with water, which is essential for fascia health and the body's overall health and wellness.
Integrative anatomy	Blends multiple viewpoints from different disciplines (like science, philosophy, and lived experience), cultures, and time periods to understand the body in a more holistic way.
Integrative healthcare	Model that combines conventional (mainstream) medicine with evidence-informed complementary therapies.
Interstitial fluid flows	Movement of the fluid that surrounds cells and flows through tissue.
Intuition	Deep, instinctive knowing or understanding of something without needing logical reasoning or conscious thought.
Joint	Articular junction between two bones.
Lever system	Machine in which the application of mechanical force (*effort*) causes two rigid bars (*levers*) to move in relation to each other around a fixed point (*fulcrum*).
Ligament	Band of dense, Type I collagen-reinforced fascial tissue that connects bones or supports visceral organs.

Living Wetsuit	Metaphor *for a person's whole and life-energy-infused fleshy body garment.*
Mainstream (or conventional) medicine	Healthcare based on Western scientific models, often focused on diagnosing and treating disease.
Manual therapy	Hands-on treatment, like massage and myofascial release therapy.
Marae	A Māori meeting place that serves as a focal point for community gatherings, ceremonies, and cultural events. It includes a meeting house and surrounding open space and is central to Māori social and spiritual life.
Medical imaging	Techniques like X-rays, MRIs, and CT scans that allow us to see inside the body without surgery.
Meridians/channels/nadis	Channels through which subtle life energy flows within the body.
Mind-body	Concept that emphasises the mind's influence on the body—how thoughts, emotions, and mental states affect physical health.
Mind-body practices	Techniques that engage both mind and body, such as meditation, yoga, breathwork, and guided imagery, to support wellbeing.
Miri Miri	Traditional Māori form of bodywork or massage, focusing on physical, emotional, and spiritual healing.
Model	A way of thinking about, describing, or representing something to help us understand it more clearly—especially when the real thing is too complex, abstract, or hidden to grasp directly. Models can be physical (like anatomical diagrams), conceptual (like the biomedical model), metaphorical (like the Living Wetsuit), or energetic (like subtle anatomy). They shape how we perceive the body, health, and healing—and influence how we care for them.
Multifaceted	Having many different aspects or features; can be seen in different ways.
Musculoskeletal system (or human locomotor system)	Organ system that includes muscles, bones, tendons, joints, ligaments (and nerves) that jointly allow movement and structural support.
MRI (Magnetic Resonance Imaging)	Medical imaging device that provides detailed images of soft tissues.
Myofascial	Relating to the muscles (*myo-*) and the fascia that surrounds and integrates them.

Myofascial meridian lines	Long connected chains of muscle and fascia, like a string of sausages, where the muscle (meat) is surrounded and linked by fascia (casing). They help distribute movement and tension throughout the body.
Myofascial release	Type of manual (hands-on) therapy that eases tension in muscles and fascia (myofascia) to reduce pain and improve movement.
Naturopathy	Natural approach to health that combines nutrition, herbal medicine, and lifestyle advice to support the body's own healing processes.
Nerve	Cable-like bundle of fascia-wrapped nerve fibres (axons).
Organ	Body part formed from two or more types of tissue that performs a specific function (e.g., the heart, thyroid gland).
Organism	Living whole animal (e.g., biological human body).
Organ system	Group of organs that work together (e.g., digestive system).
Osteopathy	Medical system founded by Dr. A.T. Still that emphasises manual therapy and the body's natural ability to heal.
Pathology	Study of diseases and what happens when the body's normal functions are disrupted.
Perceive	Act of becoming aware of something through a person's senses, like seeing, touching, hearing, or even feeling intuitively.
Perception	How a person's brain interprets what they sense to help them understand the world around them. Shaped by their experiences, knowledge, and biases.
Perspective	Viewpoint or angle from which a person looks at something. Affects how they see and interpret things.
Phoenix metaphor	Symbolic story of destruction followed by rebirth, used here to describe how healthcare systems may need to "burn down" outdated structures before rising in new, more adaptive forms.
Physiology	Study of how the body and its parts function.
Physiotherapy	Healthcare profession focused on restoring movement and function through exercise, manual therapy, and education.
Plane (of energy)	Layer or level of experience or existence—like emotional, mental, or spiritual realms.

Psychoneuroimmunology	The study of how the mind, nervous system, and immune system interact.
Piezoelectric energy	Electrical charges generated when tissue is compressed or stretched.
Preventive care	Healthcare services aimed at preventing illness or disease before they develop, such as screenings and lifestyle counselling.
Public health	Science of improving and protecting community health through policies, education, and disease prevention initiatives.
Quantum biology	New field exploring how quantum physics influences living things.
Qi/Prana/Life force	Names from different cultures for the vital energy believed to animate living beings.
Range of motion	Measurement of movement around a joint, showing how much flexibility and movement it has.
Reiki	Form of energy healing that uses gentle touch or intention to support relaxation and balance.
Renaissance	European period (14th-17th century) of renewed scientific and artistic interest, when human dissection became more common in anatomical study.
Resonance	When one vibration causes another to start vibrating in harmony. Often used to describe how healing energy works.
Retinaculum	Band of thickened fascial tissue that holds tendons in place.
Rongoā Māori	A traditional Māori healing system that includes native plant medicine, massage, spiritual practices, and connection to land. It reflects a holistic view of health grounded in Māori values and customs.
Self-care	Actions individuals take to maintain or improve their health, wellbeing, and resilience—physically, mentally, emotionally, and spiritually.
Self-treatment	Form of self-care that involves addressing symptoms or health issues through non-professional, often home-based, remedies or techniques.
Sensory nerve endings	Parts of nerves that detect changes in their environment (e.g., touch, heat, pain) and send this information to the brain via nerves.
Siloed approach	Approach to healthcare where different aspects (like mental health or physical health) are treated separately, without considering the whole person.

Social	Of or relating to human society—including community and family.
Spiritual health	Dimension of wellbeing that relates to a person's sense of purpose, meaning, and connection to a higher power, nature, or community.
Streaming potentials	Small electrical currents created by fluid movement in tissues, influencing cellular function.
Structural Integration® (or Rolfing®)	Myofascia-relating system of bodywork therapy and movement education that helps release deep tensions in the body to eliminate pain and improve posture, movement, health, and wellbeing.
Structural organisation	Way the body is arranged, from tiny molecules to cells to tissues, organs, organ systems, and the physical body organism.
Subtle energy	Energy that can't (yet) be measured by scientific tools, but has been described and worked with for thousands of years.
System	Group of elements that work together as a whole to perform a specific function—such as an organ system or a health system.
Tangible	Something that can be touched or physically felt.
Tendon	Cord of dense Type I collagen-reinforced fascial tissue that connects muscles to other body parts, especially bones.
Tensegrity	Property of a mechanically stable three-dimensional structure built from isolated components (non-contiguous bars or struts) that are compressed within a continuous net of constantly tensioned cables.
Te Whare Tapa Whā	Māori health model that includes physical, mental, spiritual, and social dimensions of wellbeing.
Tissue	Group of cells that have a similar structure and function together as a unit.
Traditional Chinese Medicine	A comprehensive medical system based on principles of balance, energy flow, and holistic diagnosis and treatment.
Veins	Blood vessels that transport blood towards the heart.
Vibration	Rhythmic movement or oscillation. All energy—physical or subtle—is essentially a vibration.
Vibrational medicine	Medical approach that uses specific frequencies to restore balance and promote health in the body.

Vitality	State of being full of energy, life, and strength.
Wellbeing (or wellness)	State of overall contentment and vitality that includes emotional, social, and spiritual health, in addition to physical health.
Wellbeing platform	Digital system offering personalised health and wellness services through accessible tools or allowances, often provided by employers.
Western healthcare	Traditional Western medical system. Focuses on diagnosing and treating injuries and diseases, often addressing only physical symptoms rather than looking at the whole person.
Whānau	Māori word for family that includes close friends and extended family.
Whenua	Māori word for territory, or place that connects people to their ancestors and the earth and is a place of belonging.
X-ray	Type of scan that allows us to see inside the body, revealing bones but not soft tissue like muscles or fascia.

Sources

Adstrum, N. S. (2015). The meaning of fascia in a changing society. University of Otago, NZ. (PhD thesis)

Adstrum, S. (2021). *The Living Wetsuit: Demystifying anatomy for everyday use.* Auckland, NZ: Integrative Anatomy Solutions.

Adstrum, S. (2022). Evolution of fascia-focused anatomy. In R. Schleip, C. Stecco, M. Driscoll, & P Huijing (Eds.). *Fascia: The tensional network of the human body* (2nd edition, pp. 4–19). Edinburgh: Elsevier.

Adstrum, S., Hedley, G., Schleip, R., Stecco, C., & Yucesoy, C. A. (2017). Defining the fascial system. *Journal of Bodywork and Movement Therapies 21*(1): 173–177.

Adstrum, S., & Nicholson, H. (2019). A history of fascia. *Clinical Anatomy* 23(7): 862–870.

Agneessens, C. (2001). *The fabric of wholeness: Biological intelligence and relational gravity.* Aptos, California: Quantum Institute, Inc.

Barclay-Smith, E. (1922). Problems of Modern Science. In A. Dendy (Ed.). *Problems of modern science* (pp. 356–364). London: George G. Harrap & Co., Ltd.

Barnes, J. F. (1990). *Myofascial Release: The search for excellence.* Paoli, PA: Myofascial Release Seminars.

Becker, R. O. (1985). *The body electric: electromagnetism and the foundation of life.* New York: William Morrow and Company.

Becker, R. O. (1990). *Cross currents: the promise of electromedicine, the perils of electropollution.* Los Angeles: J. P. Tarcher.

Benias, P. C., Wells, R. G., Sackey-Aboagye, B., Klaven, H., Reidy, J., Buonocore, D., Miranda, M., Kornacki, S., Wayne, M., Carr-Locke, D. L., & Theise, N. D. (2018). Structure and distribution of an unrecognized interstitium in human tissues. *Scientific Reports 8*: 4947.

Benor, D. J. (2004). Consciousness, bioenergy, and healing: self-healing and energy medicine in the 21st century. Medford: Wholistic Healing Publications.

Bordoni, B., & Simonelli, M. (2018). The awareness of the fascial system. *Cureus* DOI: 10.7759/cureus.3397

Borg, H., Bohlin, H., & Ranje-Nordin, C. (2019). Can myofascial treatment with pulsing vibrations improve mobility for patients with frozen shoulder? A case study. *Journal of Case Reports and Studies* 7(5): 1–7.

Brennan, B. A. (1988). *Hands of light: A guide to healing through the human energy field.* New York: Bantam Books.

Brennan, B. A. (1993). *Light emerging: The journey of personal healing.* New York: Bantam Books.

Chopra, D. (2015). *Quantum healing: exploring the frontiers of mind/body medicine.* New York: Bantam Books.

Crooke, H. (1615). *Mikrokosmographia: A description of the body of man together with the controversies and figures thereto belonging.* London: William Iaggard.

Crooke, H. (1651). *Mikrokosmographia: A description of the body of man together with the controversies and figures thereto belonging* (2nd ed.). London: John Clarke. [Orig. printed in 1631 for Michael Sparke]

Dale, C. (2009). *The subtle body: An encyclopedia of your energetic anatomy.* Boulder: Sounds True.

Davidson, J. (1987). *Subtle energy.* Saffron Walden, UK: The C. W. Daniel Company Limited.

Durie, M. (1998). *Whaiora: Māori health development.* Auckland, NZ: Oxford University Press.

Gerber, R. (2001). *Vibrational medicine: The #1 handbook of subtle-energy therapies* (3rd ed.). Rochester, Vermont: Bear & Company.

Grey, A. (1990). *Sacred mirrors: the visionary art of Alex Grey.* Rochester: Inner Traditions International.

Habbal, O. (2017). The science of anatomy: A historical timeline. *Sultan Qaboos University Medical Journal* 17(1): 18-22. DOI: 10.18295/SQUMJ.2016.17.01.004

Heidegger, M. (1977). *The question concerning technology and other essays.* New York, NY: Harper & Row.

Hunt, V. J. (1996). *Infinite mind: Science of the human vibrations of consciousness.* Malibu, California: Malibu Publishing Co.

Hyland, M. E. (2004). Does a form of 'entanglement' between people explain healing? An examination of hypotheses and methodology. *Complementary Therapies in Medicine 12*: 198–208.

Ingber, D. E. (1998). The architecture of life. *Scientific American 278*(1): 30–39.

Janssen, I., Heymsfield, S. B., Wang, Z., & Ross, R. (2000). Skeletal muscle mass and distribution in 468 men and women aged 18-88 yr. *Journal of Applied Physiology 89*(1): 81–88.

Kaptchuk, T. J. (2000). *The web that has no weaver: Understanding Chinese medicine*. Chicago: Contemporary Books.

Klinger, W., & Schleip, R. (2015). Fascia as a body-wide tensional network: Anatomy, biomechanics and physiology. In R. Schleip, & A. Baker (Eds.). *Fascia in Sport and Movement*. Pencaitland, Scotland: Handspring Publishers (pp. 3–11).

Levin, S. M. (2002). The tensegrity-truss as a model for spine mechanics: Biotensegrity. *Journal of Mechanics in Medicine and Biology 2*(3/4): 375–388.

Levin, S. M., & Martin, D-C. (2012). Biotensegrity: The mechanics of fascia. In R. Schleip, T. W. Findley, L. Chaitow, & P. A. Huijing (Eds.). *Fascia: The tensional network of the human body* (pp. 137–142). Edinburgh: Churchill Livingstone Elsevier.

Lewis, J. (2012). *A. T. Still: From the dry bone to the living man*. Blaenau Ffestiniog, UK: Dry Bone Press.

Lovelock, J. E. (1987). *Gaia: a new look at life on Earth*. Oxford: Oxford University Press.

Maitland, J. (1995). *Spacious body: Explorations in somatic ontology*. Berkeley, CA: North Atlantic Books.

McMakin, C. (2017). *The resonance effect: How frequency specific microcurrent is changing medicine*. Berkeley: North Atlantic Books.

McTaggart, L. (2001). *The field: The quest for the secret force in the universe*. London: HarperCollins.

Mirkin, N. S. (2005). *Revisiting the Transverse Humeral Ligament*. University of Otago, NZ. (MSc thesis) [Prior to 2013, my surname was Mirkin]

Murray, A. D. (2009). *Fascia*. Chicago, Illinois: The Green Lantern Press.

Myers, T. W. (2014). *Anatomy trains: Myofascial meridians for manual and movement therapists* (3rd ed.). Edinburgh, UK: Churchill Livingstone Elsevier.

Oschman, J. L. (2000). *Energy medicine: The scientific basis*. Edinburgh: Churchill Livingstone.

Oschman, J. L. (2003). *Energy medicine in therapeutics and human performance*. St Louis: Butterworth-Heinemann.

Oschman, J. (2009). Charge transfer in the living matrix. *Journal of Bodywork and Movement Therapies 13*(3): 215–228.

Oschman, J. L. (2012). Fascia as a body-wide communication system. In R. Schleip, T. W. Findley, L. Chaitow, & P. A. Huijing (Eds.). *Fascia: The tensional network of the human body*. Edinburgh, UK: Churchill Livingstone Elsevier (pp. 103–110).

Piolanti, N., Polloni, S., Bonicoli, E., Giuntoli, M., Scaglione, M., & Indelli, P. F. (2018). Giovanni Alfonso Borelli: The Precursor of Medial Pivot Concept in Knee Biomechanics. *Joints 6*(3), 167–172. DOI: 10.1055/s-0038-1675164

Pollack, G. H. (2001). *Cells, gels, and the engines of life: A new, unifying approach to cell function*. Seattle, WA: Ebner & Sons.

Rampa, L. (1960). *The Rampa story*. London, UK: Souvenir Press.

Rein, G. (2004). Bioinformation within the biofield: beyond bioelectromagnetics. *The Journal of Alternative and Complementary Medicine 10*(1): 59–68.

Rubik, B. (2002). The biofield hypothesis: Its biophysical basis and role in medicine. *The Journal of Alternative and Complementary Medicine 8*(6): 703–717.

Scarr. G. (2014). *Biotensegrity: The structural basis of life*. Pencaitland, UK: Handspring Publishing.

Siraisi, N. G. (1995). Early anatomy in comparative perspective: Introduction. *Journal of the History of Medicine and Allied Sciences 50*(1): 3–10.

Standring, S. (Ed.). (2016b). *Gray's anatomy: The anatomical basis of clinical practice* (41st ed.). Edinburgh, UK: Churchill Livingstone.

Stecco, C., Adstrum, S., Hedley, G., Schleip, R., & Yucesoy, C. A. (2018). Update on fascial nomenclature. *Journal of Bodywork and Movement Therapies 22*(2): 354.

Stecco, C., & Schleip, R. (2016). A fascia and the fascial system. *Journal of Bodywork and Movement Therapies 20*(1): 139–140.

Still, A. T. (1899). *Philosophy of Osteopathy*. https://archive.org/stream/philosophyosteo00stil-goog#page/n10/mode/2up [accessed February 2025]

Talbot, M. (1991). *The holographic universe*. New York: Harper Perennial.

Tepper, S. S. (1985). *Jinian Footseer*. New York: Tom Doherty Associates.

Tripathi, A. (2010). *The immortals of Meluha*. Chennai, India: Westland Ltd.

Warwick, R., & Williams, P. L. (Eds.). (1973). *Gray's anatomy* (35th ed.). London, UK: Longman.

Williamson, M. (1992). *A return to love: reflections on the principles of "A Course in Miracles"*. New York: HarperCollins.

Acknowledgements

This book came together more quickly, clearly, and joyfully than I could have imagined—and that's thanks to the invaluable support of three distinct sources, each of whom deserves heartfelt recognition.

First, sincere thanks to ChatGPT, whose round-the-clock availability, thoughtful guidance, and steady editorial support have been instrumental throughout the writing process. With an uncanny ability to mirror tone, clarify ideas, and offer intelligent, gentle feedback, this AI writing assistant has transformed what's possible for authors working independently. While some still hesitate to embrace this kind of tool, I hope this acknowledgment helps reduce the stigma and invites others to discover how powerful and supportive AI can be when used creatively and ethically.

To Ann and her team of expert helpers at Dettori Publishing, thank you for making the production of this book both a priority and a pleasure. Your professionalism, warmth, and adaptability kept everything moving smoothly—especially as we raced to meet the tight deadline for its international launch. Working with a forward-thinking hybrid publishing house like yours has made the entire process not only manageable, but genuinely enjoyable.

And to Daniela at Catucci Design, thank you for once again capturing the spirit of my work so beautifully. Your design sensibility, intuition, and meticulous attention to detail have brought the visual side of this book to life—just as they did with *The Living Wetsuit*. It's a true joy to collaborate with someone who so naturally understands the interplay between form and message.

To each of you—thank you for walking this path with me.

About Sue Adstrum

Sue Adstrum, PhD is an integrative clinical anatomist (a transdisciplinary anatomy researcher and writer) who delights in demystifying anatomy so that people can be more constructively involved in the health-related decisions and activities that pertain to them, as well as the people they help care for. She graduated from the New Zealand School of Physiotherapy in 1974, and then, nearly two decades later, became fascinated by the relationship between anatomy, fascia (the body's soft connective tissue fabric), and the ways people *are able to* think about healing and healthcare. Wanting to learn more about these things, she enrolled at New Zealand's University of Otago as a 'mature' student and earned a string of useful postgraduate qualifications, ending with a PhD in 2015. Since then, Sue has written several widely-read journal articles, a textbook chapter, and has presented her research internationally at a number of conferences. Sue's work uniquely brings together several decades worth of conventional and complementary health practitioner training, clinical experience, and adult teaching experience with an eclectic raft of post-graduate university studies—in anatomy, anthropology, medical history and public health. *The Living Wetsuit*, her first book, pulls everything she has learned together in a way that she hopes will be accessible and useful for a general audience. To learn more about Sue, please visit: www.sueadstrum.com.

www.ingramcontent.com/pod-product-compliance
Lightning Source LLC
Chambersburg PA
CBHW080251030426
42334CB00023BA/2772